Karu:
Growing up Gurindji

Violet Wadrill

Biddy Wavehill Yamawurr

Topsy Dodd Ngarnjal

Felicity Meakins

with photographs by Penny Smith and Brenda L Croft

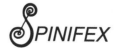

SPINIFEX

First published by Spinifex Press, 2019

Spinifex Press Pty Ltd
PO Box 5270, North Geelong, Victoria 3215
PO Box 105, Mission Beach, Queensland 4852
Australia

women@spinifexpress.com.au
www.spinifexpress.com.au

Editing: Gurindji text: Erika Charola. English text: Cheryl Leavy, Penny Smith and Erika Charola.
Editing in-house: Susan Hawthorne and Pauline Hopkins.
Back cover art: Theresa Yibwoin.
Cover design and Typesetting: Deb Snibson and Emma Statham.
Typeset in Adobe Garamond Pro
Printed by McPherson's Printing Group

Map drawn and used with permission from Brenda Thornley. Photos taken by and used with permission from Penny Smith, Brenda L Croft, Peggy Macqueen, Felicity Meakins, Justin Spence, Jenny Green, Bruce Doran, Bob Gosford, Tom and Marie Tarrant, and Ian Morris.
Front cover image: Chloe Algy and Becky Peter showing *kupuwupu* 'lemon grass' from Cattle Creek Station in 2010 (Peggy Macqueen, 2010). Back cover image: Family group at Lawi (Theresa Yibwoin, 2016).

NATIONAL
LIBRARY OF AUSTRALIA

ISBN: 9781925581836 (paperback)
ISBN: 9781925581867 (ebook: epub)
ISBN: 9781925581843 (ebook: pdf)
ISBN: 9781925581850 (ebook: kindle)

We gratefully acknowledge the support of the following organisations for their contributions to this book, and the several projects that contributed to its development.

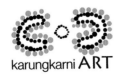
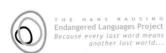
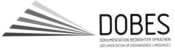
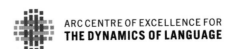

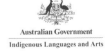

Contents

Karu: Growing up Gurindji v

Dedication vi

Preface vii

    Gurindji Language and Culture series vii

    How we made the book vii

Contributors ix

Introduction xiv

Ngarturr (Pregnancy) 1

    Karungkarni — The place of the children 2

    Yimaruk or wipilirri — Returned souls 7

    Wartiwarti karu — Born left-handed 9

    Punyu mangarri ngarturr-ku — Good foods for pregnant women 10

    Jamuny — Pregnancy taboo foods 11

Ngitji karu-wu (Caring for children) 19

Introduction 20

    Ngamayi kamparnup — Treating mothers after birth 21

    Ngapulu kamparnup — Promoting milk 22

    Karu kamparnup — Treatments using termite mound 23

    Karu kamparnup — Treatments using termite mound 25

    Warra karu parntawurru — Looking after babies' backs 28

    Purntunarri kamparnup — Treating older babies 29

    Yarnanti rarraj-ku — A charm for running 31

    Ngarrka karu-walija — Introducing children to country and ancestors 32

    Manyanyi and marlarn — Bush vicks and river red gum 34

Yarnanti kulykulya-wu — A charm for colds 35

Punyukkaji kulykulya-wu — Cures for colds 35

Yirrijkaji, wariyili and partiki — *Dodonaea polyzyga, Senna spp., Terminalia arostrata* 37

Nganany karu-wu — Warnings for children 38

Jarrakap — Learning to talk 39

Janyarrp — Baby talk 39

Jaru karu-wu — Words for babies 41

Karu yurrk (Children's stories) 45

Introduction 46

Warrija kirrawa — The crocodile and goanna 49

Ngarlkiny karu — The greedy child 55

Jajurlang — The grandmother and her grandson 63

Jampurra — The cry baby 69

Luma kurrupartu — The bluetongue and his favourite boomerang 72

Story sources 76

Karu: Growing up Gurindji

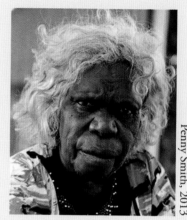

Penny Smith, 2013

Ngungantipangulu pinarrik jayinya marlurluka-lu, kajijirri-lu ngantipanguny-ju, jawiji-lu nyampa-ku, jaju-ngku, ngunyarri-lu, pinarrik mani ngungantipangulu. Wal ngurnalu ngantipa-rni nyangana ngumayijang-kulu na ngurnalu. Ngurnayinagulu ngarlaka-yirri nyamu-ngantipangulu marni ngantipanguny, jaru, jarrakap. Wal ngurnayinangulu kayi na panana ngantipa-ma, nyarrulu na, nyamu-ngantipangulu jayinya wiitwiit.

The old people taught us everything. It was our grandfathers, grandmothers and great-grandparents who educated us. They passed it all onto us orally. As the next generation, we now hold all of this knowledge. We are following in their footsteps, following what they showed us.

– Violet Wadrill 2007

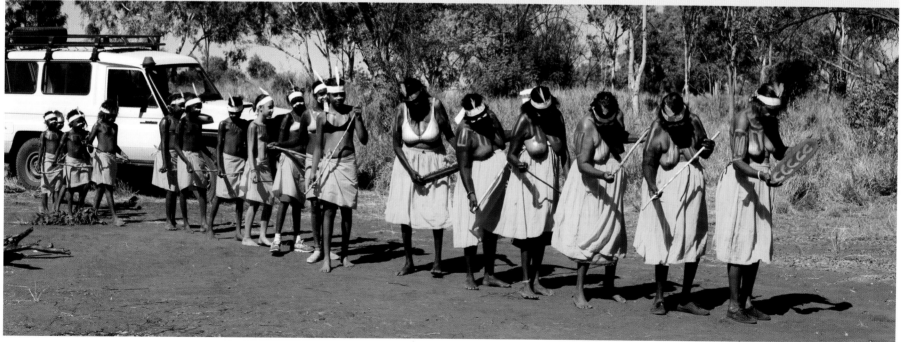

Photo: Penny Smith, 2018

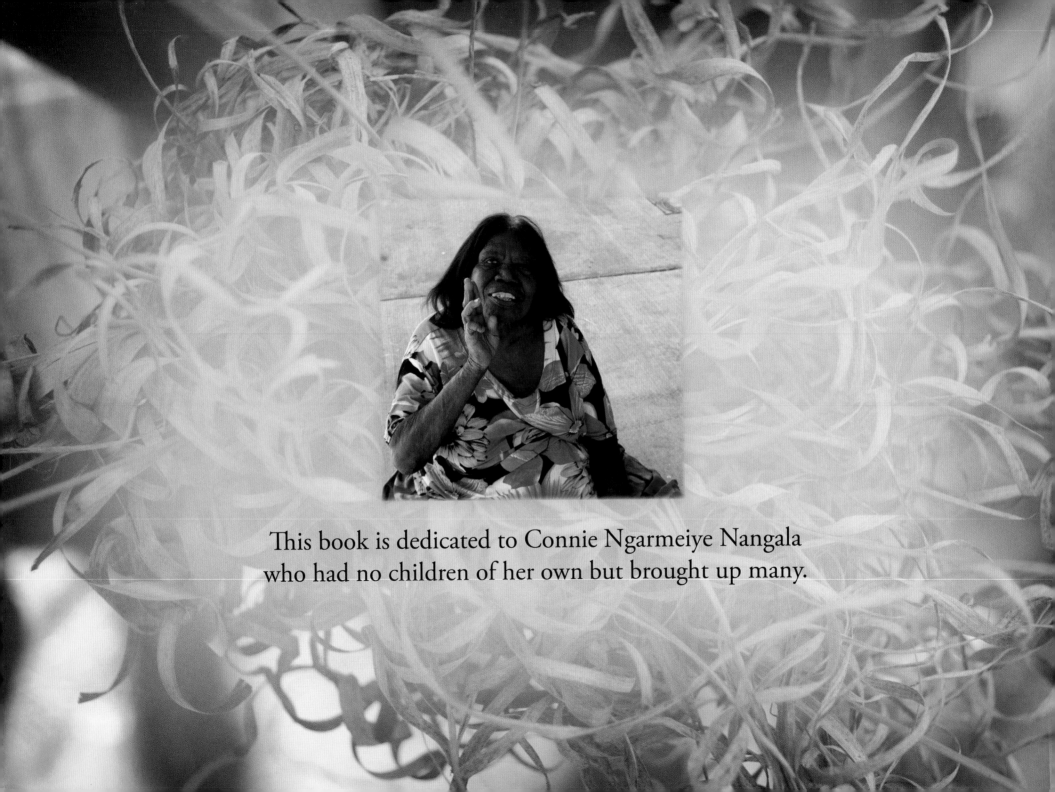

This book is dedicated to Connie Ngarmeiye Nangala
who had no children of her own but brought up many.

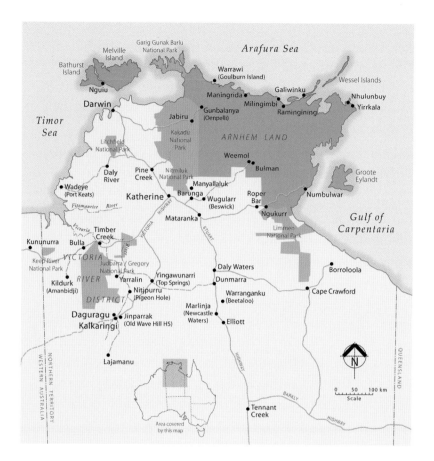

Preface

Gurindji Language and Culture series

This book is the third in the Gurindji Language and Culture series. The aim of this series is to preserve and reproduce Gurindji cultural and ecological knowledge through the Gurindji language. As Gurindji elders we believe it is important to continue passing on our knowledge to future generations of Gurindji children and to share this knowledge with *kartiya* or non-Indigenous people. Gurindji country is located in the southern Victoria River District in the Northern Territory (Australia). Most of us live on our country at Kalkaringi and Daguragu and we are best known for the Gurindji Walk-Off. This landmark event of 1966 delivered equal wages to the pastoral industry and resulted in the establishment of the Aboriginal Land Rights (Northern Territory) Act 1976.

How we made the book

Texts were produced by Violet Wadrill, Biddy Wavehill, Topsy Dodd Ngarnjal, Connie Ngarmeiye and Felicity Meakins between 2007-2018 during Gurindji language and culture documentation work. Many of the procedural texts, such as collecting and preparing bush foods and medicines, were produced as a part of contemporary everyday life. We video recorded these activities, watched the videos and made audio recordings describing the process. The description of this process was recorded in Gurindji and translated into English. Many of the videos were broadcast on ICTV (Indigenous Community Television) and are now available through their website. The production of the texts in Chapter 3 involved an art camp and is described in detail in the introduction of that chapter. Finally the charms in Chapter 2 come from Dandy Danbayarri and were recorded by Lauren Campbell. The charm texts were checked with Ronnie Wavehill by Felicity Meakins.

Images come from a number of sources. The majority of the photographs were taken by and used with permission from Penny Smith and Brenda L Croft. Permission to use images of people is with consent of the adult, or consent of the caregiver if the image is of a child. Additional photos are used with permission from Peggy Macqueen, Justin Spence, Felicity Meakins, Serena Donald, Jennifer Green, Bruce Doran, Bob Gosford, Tom and Marie Tarrant and Ian Morris. Cut out images of bush tucker and medicine were originally created for the Gurindji bird, bush medicine and bush tucker posters by Maxine Addinsall. Maps were created by Brenda Thornley.

Artworks are supplied by Karungkarni Art and Culture Aboriginal Corporation and are reproduced with permission from Theresa Yibwoin, Violet Wadrill, Serena Donald, Pauline Ryan, Rachael Morris, Sarah Oscar, Narelle Morris, Desmarie Morrison Dobbs and Rosemary Johnson. Artworks were photographed by Mick Richards.

Design The book was designed by Felicity Meakins and MAPG. English throughout the book was copy-edited by Cheryl Leavy, Penny Smith and Erika Charola, and from Spinifex Press by Susan Hawthorne and Pauline Hopkins. The Gurindji was copy-edited by Erika Charola.

Funding and support for the production of this book has come from a number of sources. Funding for the graphic design and publication of the book was sourced from the Indigenous Languages and Arts (ILA) scheme through Prime Minister and Cabinet (2014-2015, Karungkarni Art). Violet Wadrill, Biddy Wavehill, Topsy Dodd Ngarnjal and Connie Ngarmeiye and Felicity Meakins' work was financially supported by a number of grants including a Dokumentation Bedrohter Sprachen (DoBeS) grant (*Jaminjungan and Eastern Ngumpin Documentation* 2007-2010, C.I. Eva Schultze-Berndt) and an Endangered Languages Documentation Project (ELDP) grant (*The Documentation of Gurindji Kriol, an Australian Mixed Language* 2008-2010, C.I. Felicity Meakins) both administered by the University of Manchester and an Australian Research Council (ARC) DECRA (*Out of the Mouths of Babes: The Role of Indigenous Children in Language Change*, C.I. Felicity Meakins) administered through the University of Queensland. Accommodation was provided by Katherine West Health Board, Central Land Council and Kalkaringi CEC.

Contributors

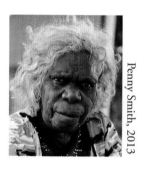

Violet Wadrill Nanaku was born in 1942. Her *kaku* (paternal grandfather's) country is Jutamaliny (Swan Yard) on Limbunya Station which is Malngin country. She grew up at the Wave Hill Welfare Settlement and Jinparrak (old Wave Hill Station) and worked on the station when she was older. She met her husband, Donald Nangka, at the station and they had seven children. Violet now lives at Kalkaringi surrounded by her 23 grandchildren and 16 great-grandchildren. She has worked extensively with Felicity Meakins, Erika Charola and Lauren Campbell on the documentation of Gurindji language and culture, including a dictionary and ethnobiology. She also paints her traditional country, Jutamaliny, and makes *kawarla* (coolamons) and *kurturu* (nullanullas). Two of her artworks are currently touring nationally as part of the exhibition, *Still In My Mind: Gurindji Location, Experience and Visuality*. She was also a finalist in the 2018 National Not-For-Profit Digital Technology Award for Story Telling.

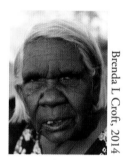

Biddy Wavehill Yamawurr Nangala was born in 1942 at Jinparrak. She grew up at the station and worked in the stockmen's quarters when she was a young woman. She met her husband, Jimmy Wavehill Ngawanyja, at the station, and they worked on many cattle stations before returning to Limbunya. They now live at Kalkaringi with their ten children, 24 grandchildren and 15 great-grandchildren. Biddy has been heavily involved with Gurindji language and culture documentation projects with Felicity Meakins, Erika Charola and Lauren Campbell. She is also a Director of the Karungkarni Art and Culture Aboriginal Corporation. She paints her Dreamings including *ngawa* (water), *janginyina* (lightning), *wampana* (spectacled hare wallaby) and *yarrkankurna* (white cockatoo). In 2011, Biddy represented the region in the development of designs for the Katherine Region Cultural Precinct, and in 2013, Biddy represented Karungkarni Art at Megalo Printmaking Studios in Canberra. Her artwork *Jinparrak* is currently touring nationally in the exhibition, *Still In My Mind: Gurindji Location, Experience and Visuality*.

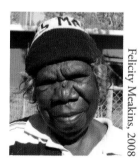

Topsy Dodd Ngarnjal Nangari was born at Jinparrak (old Wave Hill Station) in 1934. As a young woman, she worked in the stockmen's quarters serving food and washing up. She met her husband, Victor Vincent, at the station. In 1966, Victor's father, Vincent Lingiari, initiated a workers' strike to protest against the poor conditions of their employment and ultimately recover control of their traditional lands. During this period, Topsy and her husband worked at Kalkaringi which was a welfare settlement. Here she cooked for the school children. Later they moved to Jamangku (new Wave Hill Station) where she continued working as a cook and her husband worked as a stockman. Today Topsy lives at Kalkaringi with her daughters. She is a senior ceremony woman, paints and makes a number of artefacts including *kawarla* (coolamons) and *kurturu* (nullanullas).

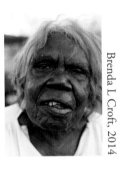

Brenda L Croft, 2014

Connie Ngarmeiye Nangala was born in 1940 to Mary Jarrngali Nangari and Joe Jumngayarri at Jinparrak under a *wanyarri* (bauhinia) and grew up at the station. She is Gurindji and Mudburra. Her *kaku* (paternal grandfather's) country is Kunawa (Cattle Creek Station homestead area) and her *jawiji* (maternal grandfather's) country is Yarri. She worked in the kitchen at Jinparrak and then worked at the police station compound at Kalkaringi where she washed and ironed clothes and did cleaning. As a young woman she was married to Clancy Parnkana and they lived at the Wave Hill Police Station. After marrying Joe Mosquito (aka Kevin Wara) she worked at Cattle Creek Station as a cook. Later she worked at Jamangku (new Wave Hill Station) and Nicholson Station also as a camp cook. She adopted two children and has six grandchildren through her adopted children. Connie is an artist at the Karungkarni Art and Culture Aboriginal Corporation in Kalkaringi and has worked with Felicity Meakins on language projects. She paints bush tucker as well as her Dreamings: *ngapa* (rain) and *wampana* (spectacled hare wallaby). One of her artworks is currently touring nationally as part of the exhibition, *Still In My Mind: Gurindji Location, Experience and Visuality.*

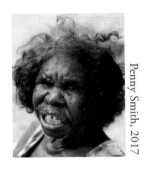

Penny Smith, 2017

Theresa Yibwoin Nangala was born in 1948 at Lipanangku to Amy Ngalngarri and Hobbles Pularranmanyu near the current Kalkaringi police station. As a young woman, Theresa lived on Wave Hill Station and her two eldest children were born there in a rock windbreak. She was one of the members of the Wave Hill Walk Off group. Her home is at Daguragu, but she now lives in Katherine so that she can receive dialysis treatment. Theresa is a member and founding Director of the Karungkarni Art and Culture Aboriginal Corporation. Her works derive from the many Dreaming stories told to her by her grandfather, Warlukirta, who was from the black soil country on Cattle Creek Station. Now these stories are in Theresa's mind and she is keen to talk about her Dreaming so as to pass on her knowledge. She is often invited to share her knowledge with Gurindji children at Kalkaringi School. Theresa paints bush tucker, such as *ngamanpurru* (conkerberry), a favourite berry which ripens after the wet season. *Ngamanpurru* is also a Dreaming for Daguragu where Theresa is a proud Traditional Owner. She is also recognised as a strong cultural knowledge holder and main custodian of many of the women's dance ceremonies.

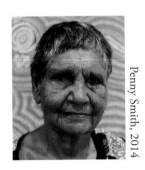

Penny Smith, 2014

Pauline Ryan Namija was born at Jinparrak (old Wave Hill Station) in 1947. As a young woman, she worked at Wave Hill and Cattle Creek Stations as a domestic servant in the dining room and men's quarters, washing and ironing. In 1966, Vincent Lingiari initiated a workers' strike to protest against the poor conditions of the employment of Aboriginal people, and ultimately recover control of their traditional land. Following the lead of Lingiari, Pauline and her husband walked off Wave Hill Station to Daguragu. They have lived in Kalkaringi since that time. Pauline started painting and sewing at Daguragu at the old Art and Craft Centre. She learned her Dreaming stories from the old people during ceremony. Pauline is a founding director of the Karungkarni Art and Culture Aboriginal Corporation. One of her artworks is currently touring nationally as part of the exhibition, *Still In My Mind: Gurindji Location, Experience and Visuality.*

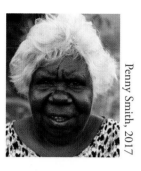

Rosemary Johnson Namija is a Warlpiri/Gurindji/Waramunga artist, and member and former director of Karungkarni Art Centre in Kalkaringi in the northern Tanami Desert/Victoria River region of the Northern Territory. Rosemary was born on old Wave Hill Station (Jinparrak) when her mother, a Waramunga woman, was working there and her father, a Warlpiri man, was working in the stock camp. Rosemary's mother was a cleaner on the station. Later she became a teacher at Lajamanu School. Rosemary lived at Jinparrak until the age of five and then grew up at Cattle Creek Station. As she grew older, she lived with her *jaju* (maternal grandmother) in Lajamanu who sent Rose to Yirarra College in Alice Springs. In 1966, at the time of the Wave Hill Walk Off, Rosemary was a little girl and was carried by her older sister as they walked to Victoria River. After the Wave Hill Walk Off, her parents moved to Lajamanu, stayed for a while and then moved back to Kalkaringi Welfare Settlement.

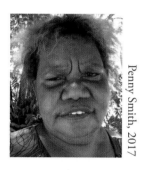

Sarah Oscar Yanyjingali Nanaku was born at Jinparrak (old Wave Hill Station) in 1964 to Josephine Nyirtungali and John Jangayarri George. She is the younger sister of Ena Oscar and was largely brought up by her. She is Gurindji and Mudburra and follows her *ngamayi* (mother's) and *jawiji* (mother's father's) traditional country which is Yamarri (Cattle Creek Outstation) and Warlujarrajarra (on Cattle Creek Station). Sarah's Dreaming is the *wayit* (pencil yam) which she paints. She is a skilled English and Gurindji translator. She is an assistant teacher at Kalkaringi school and, in her spare time, has worked with Felicity Meakins on the documentation of Gurindji language and culture. Sarah spends her weekends fishing, camping, collecting bush foods and practising bush medicine. She is passionate about continuing the traditions of her Gurindji and Mudburra ancestors. Her triptych is currently touring nationally as part of the exhibition, *Still In My Mind: Gurindji Location, Experience and Visuality*.

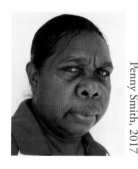

Serena Donald Larrpingali Nimarra was born in 1970 to Violet Wadrill Nanaku and Donald Nangka Jurlama in the old clinic at Kalkaringi. She grew up at Daguragu with her nine brothers and sisters and later went to school in Alice Springs. Serena is Malngin and Gurindji. Her *kaku* (father's father) country is on Riveren (Kurlungurru) and Inverway stations. Serena studied a Certificate III and IV in media at Batchelor Institute and won the Harry Wilson Memorial Award for media and radio. She has worked for the Central Land Council ranger group at Kalkaringi. She has a passion for Gurindji language and culture, and spends much of her time with Gurindji elders learning traditional stories and knowledge. On the weekends she enjoys fishing, camping and learning about the country surrounding Kalkaringi. One of her artworks is currently touring nationally as part of the exhibition, *Still In My Mind: Gurindji Location, Experience and Visuality*.

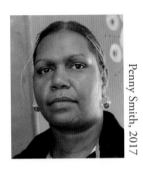

Penny Smith, 2017

Desmarie Morrison Dobbs Napurrula was born in 1989 in Tennant Creek. She grew up at Imangara (Murray Downs community). There are many artists in Desmarie's family, but she mainly learned from her mother and grandmother. Her mother and grandmother described to Desmarie how she should use certain colours to depict the landscape. Desmarie's paintings exhibit a style which derives from the distinct dot painted landscapes of the Barkly region. The paintings are often about the places and things that she did when she grew up — how to hunt, how to gather bush tucker, how to recognise the trees, plants, bush food and bush medicine. Desmarie attended Tauondi College to study art while at high school in Adelaide. Since high school, Desmarie has continued to enjoy painting as a hobby while bringing up her two young children. She recently became a member of Karungkarni Art where her works have been very popular. Desmarie has worked at the Kalkaringi Women's Safe House for seven years.

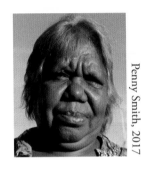

Penny Smith, 2017

Rachael Morris Namitja was born in 1963 at Jinparrak (old Wave Hill Station) to Amy Morris who was Waramunga, and Nuggett Edwards, who was Warlpiri. Rachael was three at the time of the Wave Hill Walk Off and was carried by her older sister, Helen, as they walked to their new home at Lipanangku on the Victoria River, now the site of the Kalkaringi. She later attended school at Yirrara College in Alice Springs, finishing Grade 10. During her school holidays she was able to spend time out in the bush near Lajamanu with her cousin-sister (Margaret Paddy), digging for bush potatoes, tomatoes, and onions. They also enjoyed collecting conkerberry and hunting goanna, blue tongue lizards and quolls. Rachael has been painting most of her adult life. She was a founding member of the Karungkarni Art and Culture Aboriginal Corporation in 2011 and, in its second year, she was elected as a Director. In 2012, Rachael represented Karungkarni as an Artist-In-Residence at the Songlines Gallery, Woodford Folk Festival. In 2013, she travelled to Canberra with three senior artists from Karungkarni Art as part of the 100 Years Anniversary of Canberra. In 2014, Rachael was selected by ANKAAA to participate in their Art Worker Extension Program. Her artwork is currently touring nationally as part of the exhibition, *Still In My Mind: Gurindji Location, Experience and Visuality.*

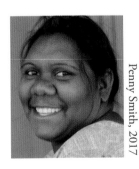

Penny Smith, 2017

Narelle (Nardia) Morris Nampin is a young Warlpiri/Gurindji artist born in 1991 in Kalkaringi. She has been an art worker at Karungkarni Art and Culture Centre since 2014. She has been a regular painter at Karungkarni Art since 2012. She loves to paint Dreaming stories, which she learnt from her mother and her grandparents. Narelle has two young children and looks after other children from her extended family. Narelle loves working at the art centre because she wants to be near the old people and listen to their stories about their Dreamings and the early days. Narelle was selected to train with IRCA (Indigenous Remote Communications Association) in Canberra and with the NT Libraries RIPIA (Remote Indigenous Public Internet Association) program in Katherine, Northern Territory to learn to record audio and visual stories.

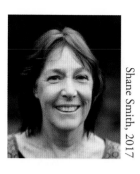

Shane Smith, 2017

Penny Smith has lived in Kalkaringi since 2011. Penny assisted local Gurindji artists in the formation of their Karungkarni Art and Culture Aboriginal Corporation in July 2011 and continued until 2019 as the manager. Penny's personal arts practice is a combination of arts project management; public art; management of festival visual art and installation; community arts workshop facilitation and hands-on multi-disciplinary arts practice. Her work also involves art and design, including illustration, illustrative mapping, photography, graphic design and book design. Prior experience includes owning and operating a successful pottery business, an art supply retail outlet, picture framing business and contemporary art gallery on Queensland's Sunshine Coast. Until February 2011, Penny was employed full-time as Visual Arts Program Manager for events organised by the Queensland Folk Federation, including the Woodford Folk Festival and The Dreaming Festival.

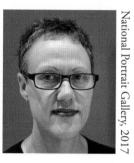

National Portrait Gallery, 2017

Brenda L Croft Nangari was born in Perth (WA) in 1964. She is from the Gurindji/Malngin/Mudburra peoples of the Northern Territory on her father's side and Anglo-Australian/German/Irish heritage on her mother's side. Brenda's father, Joseph, was born in the Victoria River region circa 1926 and his family connections are to Limbunya. In 1927, he was taken with his mother to Kahlin Compound in Darwin. In 1930 he was taken south to the Bungalow Half-Caste Children's Home and did not see his mother or family for over four decades. Brenda's family history informs her work as an artist and researcher. She has been involved in the contemporary arts and cultural sectors for three decades as an artist, arts administrator, curator, teacher, academic researcher and consultant. Brenda is an Australian Research Council Discovery Indigenous Award recipient and is completing her PhD at UNSW Art & Design. Brenda's research project *Still In My Mind: Gurindji Location, Experience and Visuality* involves working closely with her family and community at Kalkaringi and Daguragu and locations associated with Gurindji Stolen Generations members.

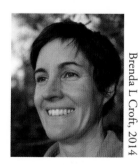

Brenda L Croft, 2014

Felicity Meakins is an Associate Professor at the University of Queensland. She is a linguist who specialises in the documentation of Australian Indigenous languages in the Victoria River District of the Northern Territory including Gurindji, Bilinarra, Malngin, Mudburra and Ngarinyman; and the effect of English and Kriol on Indigenous languages. She has worked as a community linguist with Diwurruwurru-jaru Aboriginal Corporation and as an academic over the past 19 years, facilitating language revitalisation programs, consulting on Native Title claims and conducting research into language change in Australia. She has co-compiled the *Bilinarra, Gurindji and Malngin Plants and Animals* (2012), *Gurindji to English Dictionary* (2013) and *Kawarla: How to Make a Coolamon* (2015) with Gurindji elders including Violet Wadrill, Topsy Dodd and Biddy Wavehill. She co-edited *Yijarni: True Stories from Gurindji Country* (2016) and *Mayarni-kari Yurrk: More Stories from Gurindji Country* (2016) with Erika Charola. She also co-authored *Understanding Linguistic Fieldwork* (2018) and *Songs from the Stations* (2019) with Myfany Turpin and Jennifer Green.

Introduction

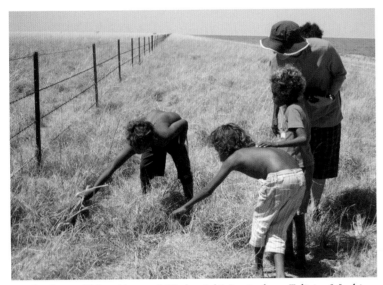

Becky Peter, Chloe Algy and Nathaniel Morris show Felicity Meakins a bluetongue burrow at Warlujarrajarra on Cattle Creek Station (Photo: Peggy Macqueen, 2010)

Much of the work in this book was foregrounded by the Aboriginal Child Language project (ACLA, University of Melbourne, 2003-2007). During this project, I partnered with a number of Gurindji mothers including Samantha Smiler, Cassandra Algy, Anne-Maree Reynolds, Ronaleen Reynolds and Cecelia Edwards to record their children, Leyton, Chloe, Byron, Tyrone and Becky, learning to speak. In the process, we documented many child-rearing practices we knew to be different from Western ways of raising children. We continued recording these customs with Gurindji elders in subsequent projects. Many of these child-rearing practices have a spiritual basis, such as why birth marks occur, the reincarnation of ancestors in utero and food taboos observed by women during pregnancy. Other cultural traditions are highly practical in nature, such as the collection, preparation and administration of bush medicines

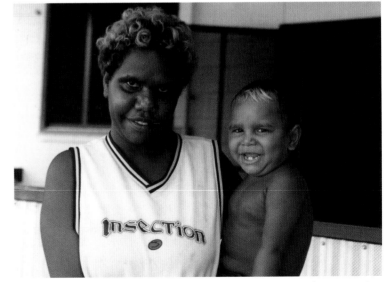

Samantha Smiler and Leyton Dodd (Photo: Felicity Meakins, 2003)

to treat children. These practices contrast with non-Indigenous child-rearing because they are deeply embedded in an understanding of country and require mothers to have an extensive knowledge of the local ecology. Yet other differences such as co-sleeping, the celebrated independence of young children and the role of older children in raising younger children are not respected as distinct cultural practices. Instead they are explicitly criticised in child health and safety campaigns, and in the plethora of non-Indigenous commentary on mothering found on social media. Some of these practices came under scrutiny in 2007 towards the end of our Aboriginal Child Language Project when the Northern Territory National Emergency Response (aka the Intervention) began under former Prime Minister, John Howard. The premise for the Intervention was alleged rampant child abuse in remote NT communities, publicised in a news story that was later found to be fabricated. While the social upheaval brought about by Indigenous dispossession has undoubtedly made for a much more challenging parenting environment for Gurindji families, there is an unfortunate re-framing of many Indigenous child-rearing practices as neglect. This contributes to the justification of the alarmingly high rate of removal of children from their families, including some of the children in our project. In most cases, the removals have been shown to be much more detrimental to the development of children than any problems faced in their home situation. The aim of this book is to re-present Gurindji child-rearing practices from an Indigenous perspective, honour those Gurindji mothers, grandmothers, assistant teachers and health workers who dedicate their lives to shaping children's lives, and to celebrate children growing up Gurindji.

– **Felicity Meakins**

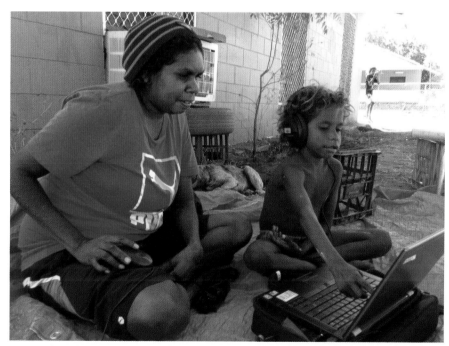

Cassandra Algy runs a rhyming game with Keithan Barry at Daguragu
(Photo: Felicity Meakins, 2015)

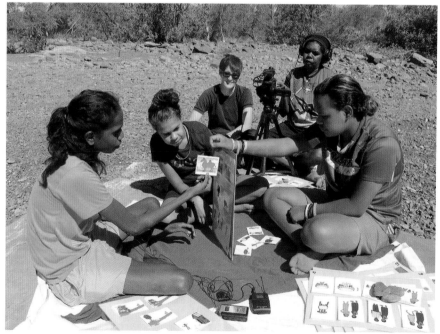

Cassandra Algy and Felicity Meakins record language games
with Jamieisha Barry, Regina Crowson and Quitayah Frith
(Photo: Jennifer Green, 2017)

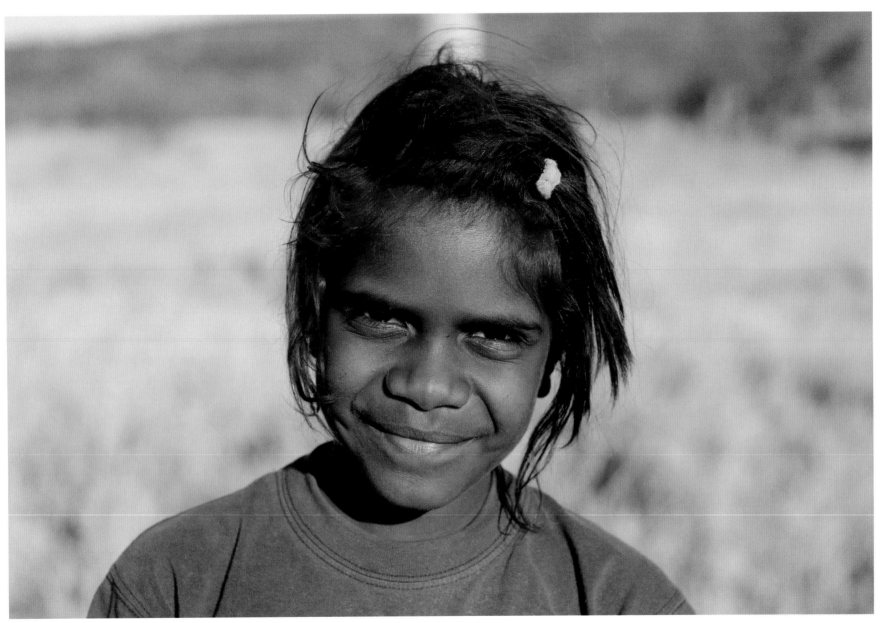

Jasmine Jimmy (Photo: Brenda L Croft, 2016)

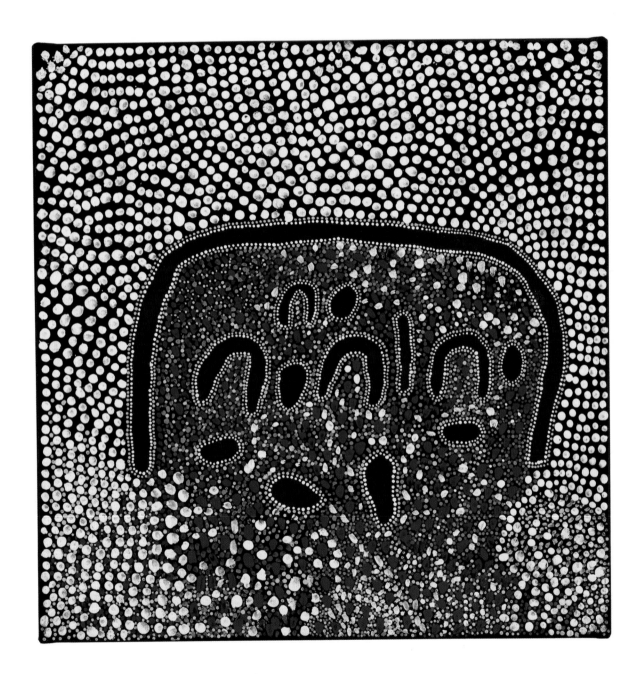

Family group (Painting: Pauline Ryan, 2017)

Ngarturr

Pregnancy

Karungkarni — The place of the children
told by Violet Wadrill

Karungkarni is a very important Dreaming hill located just south of Kalkaringi. Karungkarni Art and Culture Aboriginal Corporation is named after this hill and many Gurindji children come from this place. Prospective mothers climb the hill and brush the two Dreaming boy and girl rocks with a branch. Sometimes in the evenings, you can see the Dreaming children playing near the Victoria River at the back of the Kalkaringi rubbish dump. Violet Wadrill was told the story of the Dreaming children by her mother's sister, Ida Malyik. This version of the story was told at Jatpula.

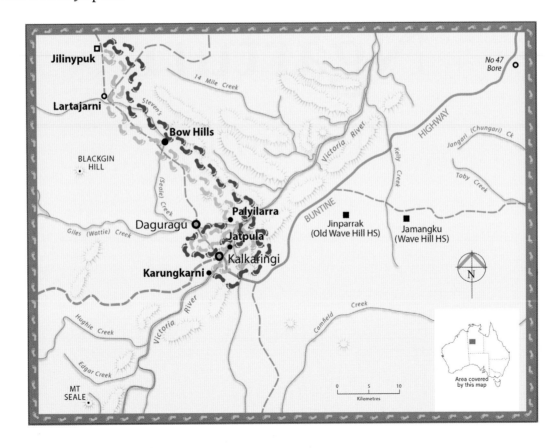

Kayiliin-nginyi nyila-ma-lu karu-ma. Kayiliin ngulu yani Jilinypuk-mayin. Jilinypuk nyawa kayirra. Lartajarni-ngurlu karrinya. Jilinypuk-kula ngulu karrinya nyila na yatu nyamu-lu wanyjarni. Yatu, ngulu wanyjarni. Karrinya ngulu yalangka kutitijkarra. "Wanyjirrirniny-parlaa yanku? Wanyjirrirniny ngurlaa yanku?" Kutitijkarra ngulu karrinya nyawa-ma Jilinypuk-nginyi-ma-lu yani yalangkurra na nyila, yatu nyamu-rlaa manana.

This is about Dreaming children who come from the north. They came from the north through Black Gin Yard which is north of here. It's not far from Black Gin Bore. They stopped at Black Gin Yard where they left some white ochre. They stood around for a bit thinking about which way to go. "Which way should we go next? Where should we go next, do you think?" said the Dreaming children. They stood about, and then from Black Gin Bore, they went to where we get white ochre.

Yalangka na ngulu kutitij-karra karrinya.
Kutitijkarra.
    "Wayi-rlaa wart yanku wayi?"
    "No, yikili na ngurlaa."
    "Kula-rlaa yanku, kayirra-ma lurrpu-ma."
    "Nyawa na ngurlaa yikili."
Nyawa ngulu yani kayiliin.

Yalanginyi-ma yatu na ngulu wanyjarni nyila-ma. Yatu, ngurnalu manana nyila-ma yatu well, nyila-ma nyamu-lu kutitij nyarrulu-ma karrinya. Ngulunyunukurla nyampayirla mani, karu-ngku-ma yalungku-ma. Wanyjarni ngulu yatu na. Nyila-ma-kata kayirra. Kutitijkarra ngulu karrinya warrij na ngulu yani yalanginyi. Kayiniin ngulu yani nyawa Bow-Hill-jirri.

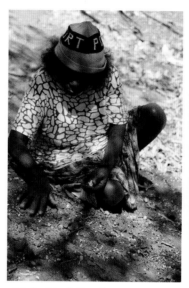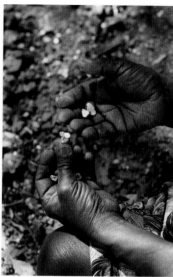

Violet Wadrill collects *yatu* (white ochre) at Latajarni
(Photo: Brenda L Croft, 2016)

There they lingered for a while longer. They were standing there thinking about which way to go.
    "Shall we go back?"
    "No we're too far away now."
    "We can't go back north."
    "We are too far away at this stage."
They had come from the north.

So they left some white ochre there. We get white ochre from where they were standing around. They left some white ochre there in the north. They hung around for a bit and then left. Then they went from the north to Bow Hill.

Bow Hill-la ngulu karrinya.
　"Ah lawara."
　"Yanku-rlaa!"
　"Yanku-rlaa warrij nyawa-ngurlu-ma."
　"Kurlarra nganayirla-yirri Palyilarra-yirri."
Kayiniin ngulu yani palangari olawei kayirrangkarra nyawa na.

They were at Bow Hill.
　"Hmm nothing's happening here."
　"Well let's go!"
　"Let's go from here!"
　"South to Palyilarra."
From the north they kept going along the north side of the black soil plain.

Winyji-ka na kayirrangkarra ngulu waninya Palyilarra-la.
Yalangarna ngulu karrinyani. Karrinyani ngulu yalangka-ma
karrinyani ngulu. Karrinyani Palyilarra-la-ma ngulu karrinyani
ngajik. Tirritirrip ngulu karrinyani. Kujarra-kari-ma-wula
wuruly-ma yani martukuja, malyju. Wuruly ngulu yanani,
yalangurlung-ma jarrwa-ngurlung-ma.

Yalangka na nguwula nyawa ngurra-ngka ngantipanguny-ja karlarra kuya
nyila. Yalangarna nguwula karrinyani wajarrap nganta-wula karrinyani
yalangka-ma. Ngurra-ngka-ma yalangka-ma ngantipany-ja-ma karlarra
kuya-ma. Wajarrajarra nguwula karrinyani. Yanani nguwula lurrpu nganta
kayirrangkarra. Yalanginyi-ma, karlarra wulngarn-ma-wula nyangani,
tarak-ma. Lurrpu nguwula yanani kayirrangkarra.

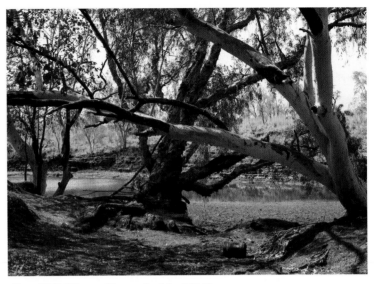

Bow Hill (Photo: Penny Smith, 2018)

They came down to a spring on the north side of
Palyilarra. Then they sat around there for a bit. They
stayed there for a while. They stayed at Palyilarra for
quite a while, camping out there. Two of the children
snuck away together — a girl and a boy. They snuck off
from the big group of children.

The two children stayed around a place a small way
west of Kalkaringi. They played about there for a
bit. Then they returned north and went down to the
spring. They saw that the sun was going down in the
west which is why they went back to the north side
of the river.

Karrinyani nguwula. Winyji-kurra yanani nguwula, jarrwa-ngkurra.
Yalangarna jarrwa-ngka ngulu karrinyani jarrwa-ngka-ma-lu
karrinyani yalangka-ma.
   "Wanyjirrirniny-parlaa yanku?
   "Wanyjirrirniny ngurlaa yanku warrij?"
   "Wanyjirrirniny-pa-rlaa pawu parru?"
   "Karru-rlaa kutirni yet,murlangka-ma ngurra-ngka-ma."
Karrinya-ngkula.

Kaputkaput-ma warrij nganta-wula yanani. Karu-kujarra-ma nyila-ma-wula
yanani. Kayiniin, pina-ngka pina-ngka-rni nguwula yanani. Kayiniin nguwula
yanani yalangkawu karlarra. Ngantipany-ja ngurra-ngka karlarra nyila.
Yalangarna nguwula karrinyani. Wajajarra-ma-wula karrinyani yalangka-ma.
Nguwula karrinyani wajajarra. Juny-ma karrinyani wulngarn-ma, kayirrangkarra
wart-parni nguwula yanani. Wart, makin-ku-ma-wula yanani yalangkurra-rni
Palyilarra-yirri-rni kayirrangkarra, makin-ku-ma.

Yalanginyi-ma, ngulu punpurru na yani purrp-parni na yalanginyi-ma.
Nyawa na kaarniin-ngayirra ngulu yani. Kaarniin-ngayirra ngulu yani nyawa
nganayirla-yirri tarukap. Nyawa kanyjurra. Jatpula-la. Tarukkarra ngulu waninya,
tarukapkarra na ngulu karrinya yalangka-ma. Kaarnimpa ngulu karrinya
tarukapkarra, purrp.

Then all of the children went together from Palyilarra. They went east,
then from the east they went to Jatpula and swam around. At Jatpula.
They got into the water and swam around there. They swam around
on the eastern side of the river until they'd had enough.

They went back to the spring where the big group of
children were and hung about for a bit. The two of
them stayed with the big group there for a while.
   "Which way should we go now?"
   "Which way will we go now?"
   "Which way will we persist in our travels?"
   "Let's stay here for a bit first in this country."
So they sat down all together.

Early in the morning, the same two children left
them again. They travelled from the north, back to
the same place in the west. Just west of Kalkaringi.
The two of them played there for a while. They kept
playing. The sun went down and they returned to the
north side of the river. They went right back north to
Palyilarra to sleep.

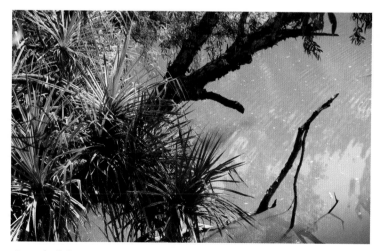

Jatpula (Photo: Penny Smith, 2018)

Kankularra warrijwarrij na ngulu yani. Kankula na, warrij nyawa na ngulu yani. Kankula ngulu yani yalangkurra-ma ngarlaka-yirri-ma. Binij mamungkul ngulu waninya yalangka-rni na. Nyila-kata punpurru kujarra-ma, martukuja, malyju. Nyila na nguwula ngajik-parni na mamungkul waninya. Nyila-ma kayiliin-nginyi, nyamu-wula yani. Dats all marntaj kuya na.

They headed upwards. Up and up they went. They went up the hill there called Karungkarni. That's where they stayed for good, turning into Dreaming features. Right there is where the two of them are — the female and male child. Those two turned into a Dreaming feature permanently. That's the story about the two children who came from the north!

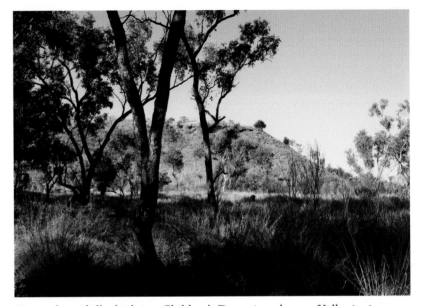

Karungkarni hill which is a Children's Dreaming close to Kalkaringi (Photo: Penny Smith, 2017)

Yimaruk or wipilirri — Returned souls

told by Biddy Wavehill with Violet Wadrill

Nyamu-lu yanana karu-yu na nyampayirla wipilirri like when they get 'em might be barramundi or might be kirrawa ngulu panana, and that karu im ngamayi blanga im mother na, kuya. We call 'em like kuya-ma 'wipilirri'. Yani nyila-ma karu-ma ngu manyirrkila manyirrkila like barramundi wipilirri na wipilirri dat karu we call 'em 'wipilirri'. Like nyanuny-ju ngaji-ngku where im kill 'em that might be barramundi or might be kirrawa, anything, snake, well that karu comes back for nyanuny ngamayi kuya. And you look that karu might be im broken one kuyany. Kuya nawun you know. And when im jarrwaj karna-ngku kuya. We call 'em 'wipilirri'.

A child spirit enters a prospective mother when her husband kills a barramundi or goanna, for example. We call that child a 'wipilirri' (or 'yimaruk') which is a returned soul. If a husband catches a barramundi, goanna or a snake — anything really — its spirit can enter the woman's belly. If you see the baby has a crooked finger, dimple, harelip or a birthmark of some kind, you know that's where the father speared the animal.

Nyila-ma nyamu-rnangku yurrk kuya-rni. Nyamu-lu panana, manyirrkila, ngaji-ngku nyanuny-ju, wal, ngurla ngamayi marnana nyanuny-ku ngamayi-yu-warla. Nyila-ma nyangana ngu nyampayirla-ma manyirrkila-ma yalangku-ma kirri-ngku-ma nyanuny-ju-ma paku yuwanana. "Nyampawu-ja-n yijkurrp yuwani?" Im know nyanuny-ju ngumparna-lu. "Ah might be karu." Ah karrinyana ngajik-piya ngarturr na." Well nyila-ma karu-ma nyamu waninyana paraj-ma. Waninyana na ngurla nyangana na nyampa-ku-rla nyawa-ma nyanawu nyamu-lu pani manyirrkila. Kamparrijang-kulu-ma they bin tell 'em you know. Kuya, marntaj.

This is what I'm telling you. As she starts to eat the barramundi and vomits, he knows she's pregnant (because the child — the 'wipilirri' — is tickling her inside). "Why are you vomiting?" Her husband knows then that she is pregnant. She will have been pregnant for a little time now. When the baby is born, they see a mark and know it was a 'wipilirri' from the barramundi. The old people always described conception like this. For example when my grandson Lee was in his mother's tummy, his father Damuel Jimmy caught a baby crocodile and kept it in a jar. It made a 'nyirt nyirt' sound. The floodwaters came up and took the crocodile away in 2001 and they were evacuated to Katherine. When they came back from Katherine, Lee was born and when he slept he would make the same noise as a baby crocodile.

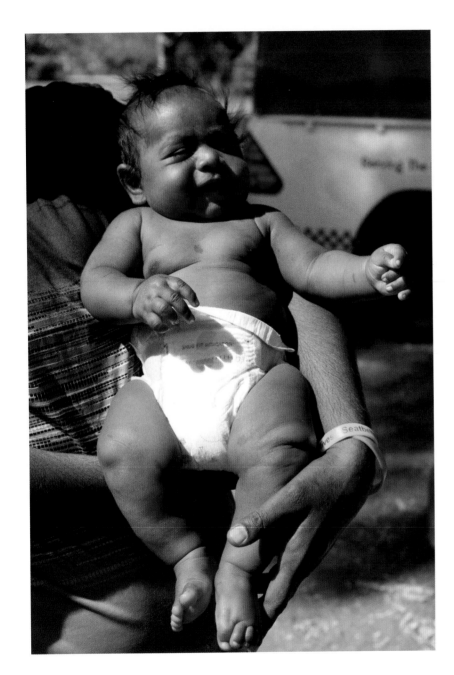

A 'yimaruk' can also be the returned soul of a family member who has passed away. Marlene Barry and Boyd George's three month old baby Luca was born with a dark birthmark around his neck and others on his torso, arms and legs. They are recognised as marks from Pamela Morris' husband who had passed away recently. (Photos: Penny Smith, 2018)

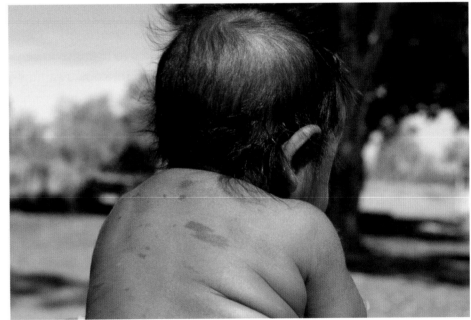

Wartiwarti karu — Born left-handed
told by Violet Wadrill with Topsy Dodd and Biddy Wavehill

Nyamu-lu-nyunu tie 'em up manana ngirlkirri when they born. Im tie 'em up mijelp kuya ngirlkirri-ma. Tingkirt manana julu-ngku kuya. Nyamu-lu waninyana karu, yapakayi, well, ngunyunu tingkirt na manana kuya julu-ngku-ma. Tingkirt ngunyunu manana. Well ngurnalu nyangana karrap kuyangku you know, yapakayi-ma nyila-ma. Ngurnalu ngarrka na manana kuyangka-ma. Nyawa-ma wartiwarti-said ngu karu-ma. Ngunyunu tingkirt manana julu-ngku kuya. Kuya na.

Sometimes babies get tied up with their umbilical cords during birth. The umbilical cord can tie itself around the baby's throat. If that happens, we'll examine that little baby. We'll recognise it's left-handed. The little one's left-handed because it was born with its umbilical cord wrapped around its neck. That's how it happens.

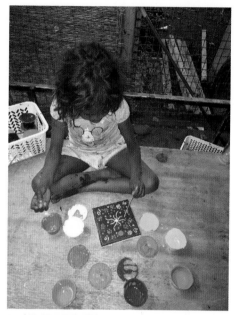

Sedonyae Donald was born left-handed. Her grandmother Serena Donald teaches her to paint and she uses her left-hand. (Photo: Serena Donald, 2018)

Punyu mangarri ngarturr-ku — Good foods for pregnant women

told by Biddy Wavehill with Violet Wadrill

Ngulu nyangani mangarri kamparrijang-kulu-ma — japawi, wutuyawung, nampula, nyilarra nyilarra, nyampayirla. Kaja-ngkurra nyamu-lu yanani nyila wayita nyampa ngulu nyangani, yangunungku, pinka-ngarna-ma nyawa-ma. Nyampayirla kinyuwurra nyampa ngulu nyangani an nyawa pinka-ngarna kanyjupal that's all, ngulu nyangani wutuyawung.

In the past pregnant women used to eat figs of different types, bush apples and more of those kinds of foods. When they went bush they would eat bush potatoes of various types and anything growing at the river. And they would eat bush onions and anything growing by the river — that's all they'd eat. Fruit and other things.

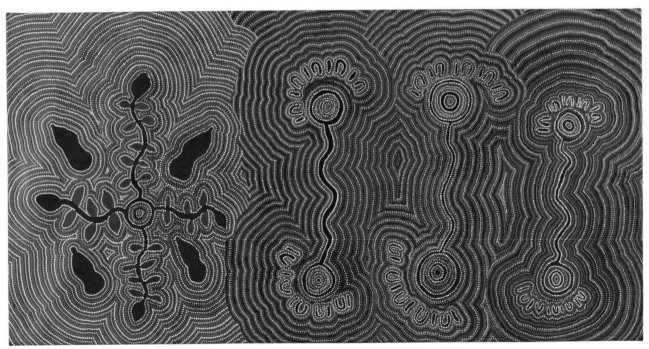

Nangari and Nanaku Women Collecting Bush Potatoes (Painting: Pauline Ryan, 2017)

Jamuny — Pregnancy taboo foods

told by Violet Wadrill with Biddy Wavehill

Kiliny — Goanna with eggs

Kula ngalu kampij-jawung-ma kirrawa-ma. Ngaja janga karrinyana karu-ma nyila-ma, ngarturr-jawung-kulu-ma. Kula ngalu. Karu-ngku ngaja karrwarnana mantara, kampij-jawung-kulu nyawa-ma. Ngulu kuya na wanyjarnani kamparrijang-kulu. Nguyinangulu marnani nganany. Kajijirri-ma, pinarri-ma. "Warta kula-n ngalu nyila-ma. Wanyjarra!" Ngurnalu ngalu ngantipa kajijirri-lu jaartkarra-ma kuyany-ma. "Kula-nta ngalu kuyany na." 'Kiliny' na dat kirrawa neim. "Kula-nta ngalu. Yarrularn-tu-ma janka-ku-ma," kuya. "Ngungantipa ngantipanguny jangkakarni-lu ngurnalu ngalu kajijirri-lu kuyany."

An expectant mother shouldn't eat gravid goannas (goannas with eggs) in case the baby gets sick. The baby might be born with sores if she does. So she can't eat it. The baby might get sores from the gravid goanna. That's why they used to leave it in the old days. They used to warn us. Those women from the old days were clever. "Hey don't eat that one," they would say. "Leave it!" Only old women could eat that one. "You mob shouldn't eat that kind of food." 'Kiliny' is the word for a gravid goanna. "Don't eat it you mob! Young women shouldn't eat it," they said. "That's only for us. Only old women can eat that kind of food."

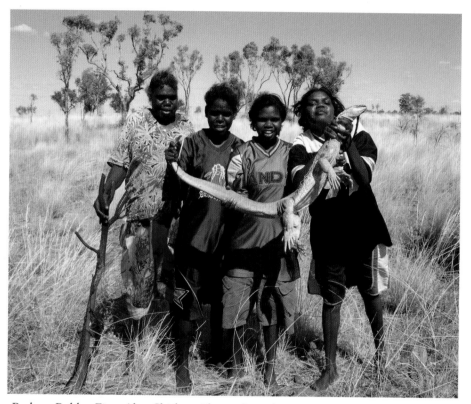

Barbara Bobby, Fiota Algy, Shirlene Algy and another young woman with a goanna at Pigeon Hole. Over the past ten years, cane toads have devastated the Victoria River District goanna population. (Photo: Justin Spence, 2007)

Jamut — Bush turkey

Jamut namata turturl-la ngulu ngarrungkap manani namata wupkarra-la, nyamu-wa jiyarni. "Wartarra wararr-jawung!" Wararr you know ngarrungkapkarra. Wararr-jawung ngurnalu ngalu. Lawara kula-n ngalu nyila-ma. Kula-ngkulu jayingku, kajikajirri-lu-ma, ngaja karrinyana ngirlkirri wankaj karu-ma. Nyila-rni karru nyamu marnana nyantu. Parrngart, ngirlkirri wankaj. Nyamu marnana, "Shhh-kaarra, nyila na. Well kuyany na ngaja karu-ma karrinyana, ngirlkirri-wu-ma, jarrakap-ku-ma. Jamut-ma im kuyany gigin karu-yawung-ku-ma, yapayapa-yawung-ku-ma.

Even if pregnant women wanted roasted turkey, they couldn't eat it when it was cooking. "Hey that's a nice fatty one". Fat is the most desirable part you know. We would want to eat the fatty meat. But you couldn't eat turkey. The old ladies wouldn't give it to you in case the baby was born with a bad throat. Turkeys make a 'shhh' sound [which you can hear when you're hunting]. It goes like this — 'shhh'. Well that's how the baby will sound when it starts to talk. That's what eating bush turkey when you're pregnant will do to you.

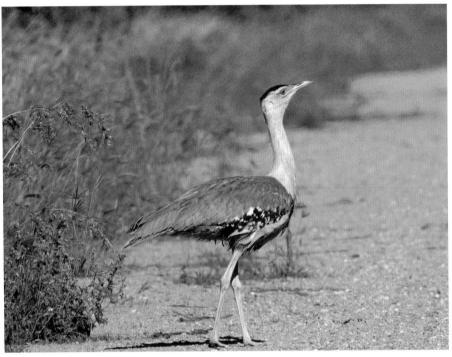

Jamut (Australian bustard, *Ardeotis australis*) (Photo: Bruce Doran)

Yiparrartu — Emu

Kula-n ngalu yiparrartu too, karu-yawung-kulu-ma, ngaja janga karrinyana yapakayi. Kuyarra-la-ma. "Wanyjarra-lu!" Kula-rnalu ngarnani kamparrijang-kulu jaartkarra-ma kuya. Nguyinangulu marnani kajijirri-ma ngaja-nta nganta ngumayijang-kulu-la. Ngaja-lu karrinyana wankaj karu. Kuya nguyinangulu marnani. Namata wararr-jawung nyamu jipij jiyarnani. Nyangani ngulu ngulu ngarramkapkarra manani you know jaartkarra-wu. Lawara, kula-nta ngalu. Ngurnalu ngalu ngantipa-rni marlurluka-lu, kajijirri-lu, jaartkarra-ma. Kula-nta ngalu, yarrulan-tu-ma kirri-ngku-ma, karu-kari-yawung-kulu-ma, wanyjarra-lu. Parik wanyjarra-lu. Kula-nta ngalu!"

You can't eat emu either if you're pregnant in case the baby gets sick. "You mob leave that [meat] alone!" So we never used to eat it in the old days. That's what the old ladies used to tell us in case it affected the next generation. Because it might cause problems for the baby. That's what they used to tell us. Even if it was a nice fatty emu cooking. The [pregnant women] used to see emu and want to eat it. "Sorry but you mob can't eat it. Only us old people can eat it. You mob can't have it. You're pregnant so you have to leave that meat. Don't have it. You mob shouldn't eat it!"

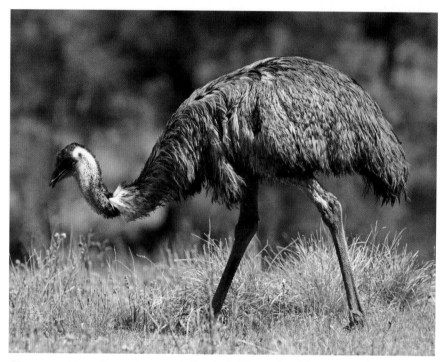

Yiparrartu (Emu, *Dromaius novaehollandiae*) (Photo: Ian Montgomery)

Narrinyjila — Turtle

Narrinyjila-ma kuya-rningan. Nguyinangulu yuwanani kamparrijang-kulu-ma nganta. Nguyinangulu yuwanani, ngaja karrinyana wankaj lanti, karu, narrinyjila-nginyi-ma. Nguyinangulu nganta marnani. "Karrurra wankaj. Nomo nganyja-lu!" Ngurnalu karu-yawung-kulu nganyja-lu. An karu-ngku yalangku kula ngalu, ngaja karrinyana wankaj lanti-kujarra, mingipkaji.

Turtle is another pregnancy taboo food. Expectant mothers used to put it aside in the old days in case the baby was born with bad hips. I think that's what they used to say. "The baby will be disabled. Don't you mob eat it!" So those of us who were pregnant would leave it. And the kids wouldn't eat it either in case they ended up crawling with two bad hips.

Wintuk — Bush stone-curlew

Nyila-ma jurlak-ma wintuk-ma-ngkula kurru karrinyani nyampayirla-lu ngarturr-jawung-kulu nyamu-yinangulu karru karrinyani. Jurlaka nyila na wurunykarraaji. Wankaj drangkarraaji. Karu-ma-lu-nga karru drangkarraaji yalanginyi-ma. Nyamu-yinangulu ngamayi-lu kurru-ma nyangana. Wankaj nyila-ma jurlak-ma. Nyantu-ma yanana ngu wurunykarra-la marnana ngu, murluwu-ma wawurru-la-ma. Yalanginyi-ma waninyana na. Jurrkjurrkkarra na karru-ma-nga. Wal kuyangka na, nyamu-lu ngarturr-jawung-kulu-ma kurru-ma nyangana yikiliyikili-ngulu jurlak kayi panana, karu-ngku-ma yalungku-ma. Nyamu-nga born manku.

A bush stone-curlew is dangerous for pregnant women to hear or be near. It whistles and moves like a drunk. Unborn babies will take after the bird. So women with small children and pregnant women can't listen to curlews. That bird is no good. It goes along whistling in the scrub. Then it falls over. It might convulse then. It will get up afterwards. Well, if the expectant mothers hear it, the babies will follow its ways [and have fits] when they're born.

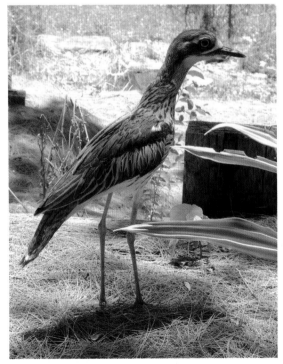

Wintuk (Bush stone-curlew, Burhinus grallarius)
(Photo: Tom and Marie Tarrant)

Jungkuwurru — Echidna

Jungkuwurru najan. Jungkuwurru-ma kula-lu ngarnani. Kuya gigin wanyjarnani ngulu. Karu-walija-lu-ma an ngamayi-lu, jungkuwurru, kula-lu ngarnani najing. Ngulu ngarnani kajijirri-lu-rni. Jangkakarni-lu-rni ngulu ngarnani. "Lawara kula-n ngalu karu-yawung-kulu-ma!" Namata tanku-murlung-kula nguyinangulu nyampayirla manani mumungku manani. Tanku-murlung-kula-ma marntaj. Mumungku manani nguyinangulu. "Kula-n ngalu," kuyangku-rni. "Ngantipa-rni ngurnalu ngalu jangkakarni-lu-rni. Nomo yapayapa-yawung-kulu, nyila-ma jungkuwurru-ma." Kuya-rni nguyinangulu mumungku manani. Marntaj.

Echidnas are also restricted for pregnant women. They didn't eat them in the old days. They had to leave that one alone too. Children and expectant mothers couldn't eat echidna. Only adults could eat it. "No, you can't eat it if you're pregnant!" It didn't matter if we were hungry, they would hold us back. And we would be hungry, OK. But they would stop us from eating it. "You can't eat it," they would say. "Only us adults can eat it. But not pregnant women." They'd say that to prevent us from eating it. That's how it was.

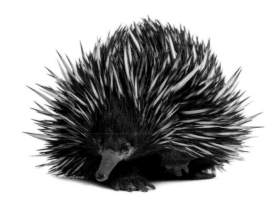

Ngapuk Ngarin — Smelling cooking meat

Kula wupkarra-la-ma nyampa-ka-ma ngapuk manku ngarin-ma ngarturr-jawung-kulu-ma. Lawara — ngaja karu nyurrun manana ngapuk-kula, majul-ta, kuya. Nyawa-ma-lu kamparrijang-kulu kuya marnana, nyamu-rnalu karrinyani kaarnimpa Jinparrak-kula-rni, kuya-rra. Jalajala rait murlangka. Ngulu kamparnana anyway-yarla murlangka-ma. Only larrpa Jinparrak-kula, kula-rnalu ngapuk manani, ngarin-ma nyampa-ma wupkarra-yirri-ma, turturlarra-yirri wupkarra-yirri, ngapuk. Ngaja karu wankaj karrinyana. Ngurnayinangulu jululuj kangani ngapuk-kula-ma, warrij, ngurla yikili ngurnalu jidan karrinyani. Lurlu-ma-rnalu karrinyani yikili karu-yawung-parni. "Warta ngurna kangana ngapuk-kula, karu! Yuu kangka-yi yalangka karru yikili-piya, ngapuk-kula-ma," kuya. "Ngaja payarru nyampa kuyany majul. Ngaja janga karrinyana. Kangka-yi kirri karrwa." Yijarni. Nyamu-lu kamparnani, nakurr-a jipij ngarin, nyila-ma-rnayinangulu karrwarnani kuya-marraj yikili nyawa purriyip maitbi kaarni in-ta purriyip-kula. Im karlarrak dat ngapuk kuya. Hmm, kuya na. Ngurnayinangulu karrwarnani karu-ma yikili.

When meat is roasting, a pregnant women shouldn't smell it. Not at all or else she might have a miscarriage. That's what they used to say in the old days when we were living right on the east side of old Wave Hill Station. Nowadays we don't worry about it so much. They cook meat any old way here. It was only in the old days at old Wave Hill Station that we couldn't smell meat roasting either in the coals or on the coals. In case the baby would get ill. The developing baby might have gotten sick. So we used to take our developing babies away from the smoke and keep our distance from the fire. When we were pregnant, we used to sit further away. "Hey I don't want the baby I'm carrying to smell it. Yes bring some food to me. I have to sit far away from the aroma of cooking meat. It might hit my belly and make the baby sick. So just keep it away from me." This is true! When they used to cook meat in the ground, we used to keep our swelling bellies a long way out of the path of the wind. The smell would go westwards. That's how things were. We used to keep our unborn babies some distance from the cooking meat.

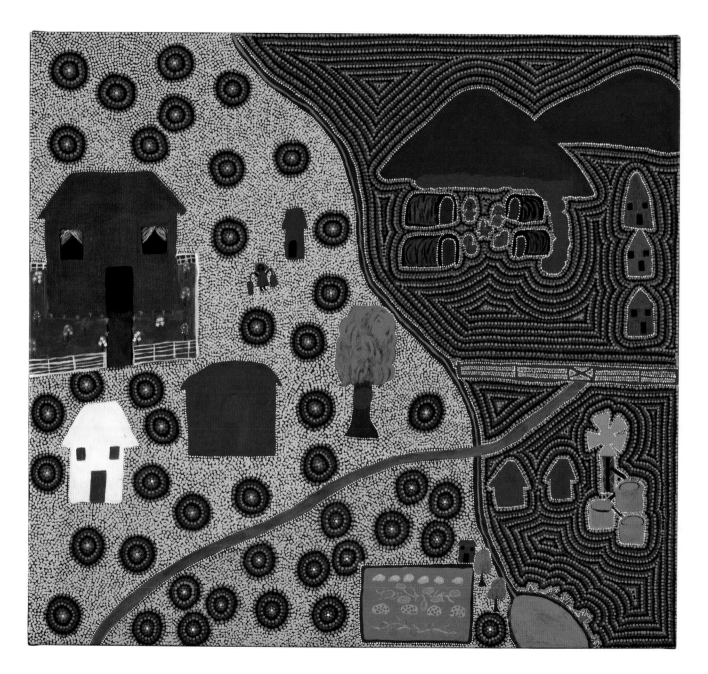

Jinparrak — Old Wave Hill Station
(Painting: Rachael Morris)

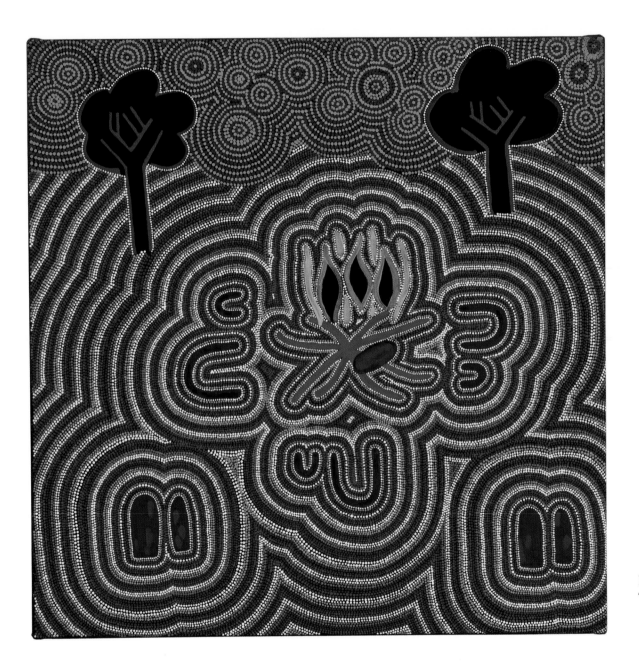

Karu Kamparnup — Treating Babies with
Termite Mound (Painting: Tara Long, 2017)

Ngitji karu-wu
Caring for children

Introduction

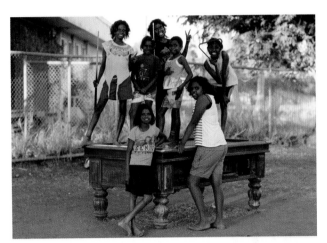

Biddy Jimmy, Jasmine Jimmy, Xaena Roy, Edwina Mick, Lukesha Jimmy and others (Photo: Brenda L Croft, 2016)

Gurindji children grow up in an ever-changing world. Continuity of tradition is coupled with the introduction of modern practices. This chapter focuses on traditional aspects of child-rearing. It begins with descriptions of various bush medicines used to treat new mothers and babies. Many of these treatments use the fine inner soil of *tamarra* — termite mound or antbed — as the base for other infusions. For example, *tamarra* is heated on a fire, crushed and mixed with *ngirirri* ash (hakea) and *ngawa* (water). Newborns are slathered with this warm mix to close their fontanelles and build up their strength. Around the age of one, babies' lower backs and knees are treated with the same mixture to strengthen their bodies for walking. Strengthening babies is a common theme. For example, coolamons are also used to keep babies' backs straight as they grow.

Other medicinal practices treat common ailments. Most of the plants used are highly aromatic, such as *marlarn* (river red gum), *kupuwupu* (lemon grass), and *manyanyi* (bush vicks). In some cases, bunches of leaves and young stems are laid on smouldering fires to create cleansing smoke which babies and toddlers are held over. Other leaves are boiled so children can be bathed in the infusion or drink the tea.

Many developmental stages are monitored to ensure that children reach important milestones. Some of these milestones are not unlike those observed the world over, such as learning to walk and talk. Other practices are unique to the region, for example fontanelle closure in young babies and the acquisition of sign language before speech. Ways of interacting with babies also can have a Gurindji flavour, such as the palatisation of 't' in baby talk. For example *karnti* 'tree' is pronounced *kanyji* when adults are talking to babies. Violet Wadrill, Biddy Wavehill, Topsy Dodd and Connie Ngarmeiye are senior Gurindji women who have brought up generations of children. In this chapter they describe ways of caring for Gurindji children, adopting and refining the practices of previous generations of women.

– **Felicity Meakins**

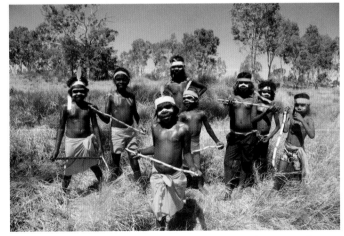

Lena George, Biddy Jimmy, Mona George, Calveena Ricky, Johneisha Ricky, Sherliyah Shaw and others painted up for dancing Freedom Day wajarra (Photo: Penny Smith, 2014)

Ngamayi kamparnup — Treating mothers after birth
told by Violet Wadrill

Nyila-ma ngu karu-nginyi kirri-ma. Karu ngu yapakaru karrwarni. An ngurnayinangulu kamparnana na tamarra-lu, ngamayi-ma. Ngirirri-lu jurrpara-lu. Kurrijkarra ngurnayinangulu pungana tarlukurruk janyja-ma. Jiyarnana strongbalak ngamayi-ma, patawankik. Ngapulu too kamparnana ngurnayinangulu nyila-ma, karu-wu na yapawurru-wu na. Kamparriijang-kulu-ma ngurnayinangulu kamparnani kuya na, Jinparrak country-ma. Turturl, jipij ngamayi-ma jiyarnani. Majul ngurnayinangulu kamparnani. An ngurnayinangulu-rla jamana ngantipanguny waninyani kuyany-ja majul-la. Tarap ngurnayinangulu kamparnani. Marntaj, kuya na.

This is how we care for women who have just given birth. We treat the new mothers with termite mound and hakea. We hollow out the ground for them and put this mixture in. The mothers get their strength back this way. Then we treat their breasts to promote their milk. This was how it was done in the old days at Wave Hill Station. The mothers would be treated this way in the warm pit. We used to heat-treat their bellies and we would put our feet on their bellies afterwards. Then we would bury them with the hot mix. That's how we did it.

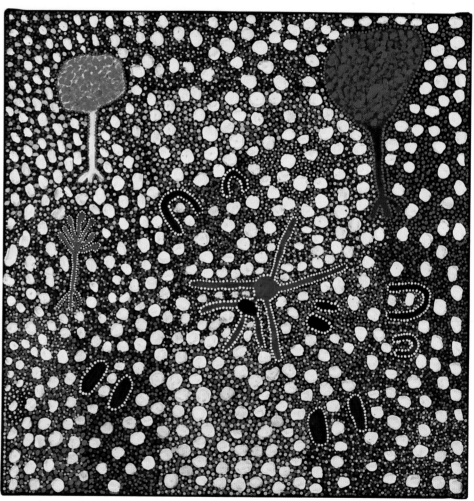

Karu Kamparnup — Treating Babies with Termite Mound
(Painting: Pauline Ryan, 2017)

Ngapulu kamparnup — Promoting milk

told by Violet Wadrill

Ngurna-rla pirrkap mani purinyjirri-la. Tamarra, tajkarra ngurna pani ngirirri-la. Ngirirri parlak. Ngurna warlu-ma pirrkap mani, ngurna-rla karu-wu-ma, kamparni ngurna. Turtul ngurna kamparni Namij. Nyanuny ngapulu. Kula ngarnani karu-ngku-ma yalungku-ma. Nyuknyukkarra ngurla payarnani ngapulu-ma. Yunyjuyunyjukkarra ngurla payarnani ngapulu-ma Nampin-tu-ma yapakaru-lu-ma. Ngurna kamparni na.

I made [the antbed treatment] in the evening to treat my granddaughter Philomena who was a new mother. I crushed the termite mound up with hakea ash. It was mixed with the hakea. I made a fire to burn the hakea to ashes and mixed it with heated-up termite mound. I heated them for the baby's milk. That baby wasn't getting any. She was suckling [but with no results]. Philomena's milk hadn't come in yet.

Makin-ta ngurna-rla pirrkap mani tarlukurru. Makin-ku tarlukurru-la na ngurna kamparni jipij, purunyjirri-la-ma. Jiyarni ngu. Ngurnayinangulu kuya na pirrkap manana tarlakurru, kamparnu-wu-ma ngapulu-wu-ma.

Turturl ngurna kamparni Namij-ma makin-jirri. Karrwi-kujarra ngurna kamparni, ngapulu an mangarri. An majul ngurna kamparni, makin-jirri warrngarlap-jirri, purinyjirri-la. Nguja kamparni ngayirra Kitty-ngku. Kuya na ngurnayinangulu kamparnana. Nyawa-murlung ngapulu-murlung-ma karrinyana karu-ma.

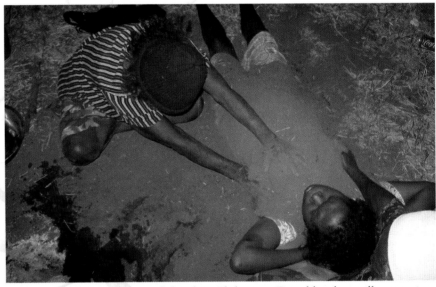

Violet Wadrill treats her grand daughter Philomena Donald so her milk comes in (Photo: Penny Smith, 2012)

I made a hollow for Philomena to lie in. I treated her while she was in the hollow in the evening. It warmed up her torso. We make hollows for new mothers like this when their milk hasn't come in yet.

While Philomena was lying down in the hollowed out fire pit, I treated her with the heated termite mound and hakea wood. I pushed it under her arms and across her breasts and chest. I also put the heated mix on her stomach while she was lying on her back. This is done for the babies who aren't getting milk.

Karu kamparnup —
Treatments using termite mound
told by Violet Wadrill

Ngurnayinangulu kamparnana karu, nyamu-lu ngajkula karrinyana, jangkakarni-wu too. Kurrij ngurnalu manana nakurr. Nakurr kurrij. Yalangarna ngurnalu yuwanana ngamanpurru, wurruja ngamanpurru, karnti. Pirrpun ngurnalu yuwanana, an ngamanpurru. Jalyi, pirrpun jalyi, yirrijkaji, marlarn. Ngurnayinangulu karu-ma kamparnana an nyawa ngurnalu yuwanana nyampayirla, warraaj. Warraaj ngurnalu kuyangku yuwanana, takurl. Jiyarnana ngapuk punyu.

We treat babies with infusions based on termite mound when they have diarrhoea — adults too. We hollow out a bit of ground and then we put in dry branches from conkerberry and turpentine bushes. We also use the leaves from *yirrijkaji* and river red gums. We treat the babies with this mixture. We often put wax in too and let the smell waft up. The lump of wax goes in among the other bush medicine in the hole. It smokes and the babies inhale it.

Ngurnayinangulu karu-ma yuwanana jarlapal kuyangku. Majul jiyanana ngu jarlapal-jirri. Yalanginyi wirrminy ngurnayingulu kuya, kankulupal, parntawurru jiyarnana ngu maru-kijak. Yalanginyi-ma ngurnayinangulu lurlu yuwanana kuya yalangka-ma tarlukurru-la-ma jungkart-ta-ma. Lurlu kuya. Kanyjuliyit-ngarna jiyanana ngu, maru-ma. Kuka-ngka-ma wankaj nyamu-wa karrinyana ngajkula-ma. Jiyarnana ngu marntaj.

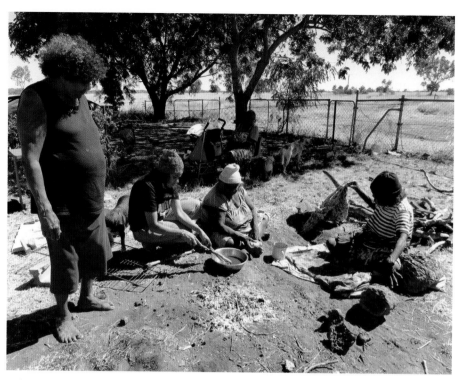

Gladys Farquarson, Leah Leaman, Kitty Mintawurr and Violet Wadrill prepare the antbed and hakea mix for Philomena Donald's daughter Sedonyae (Photo: Felicity Meakins, 2012)

We put the kids on their tummies while holding them so they can inhale the smoke. After lying them on their tummies, we turn them over and smoke their stomachs. Then we turn them over again and smoke their backs, from their bottoms upwards. Finally we sit them in the warm pit in the smoke. The smoke rises from their bottoms up. This helps them when they have bad diarrhoea.

Yalanginyi-ma jarlarlang ngurnayinangulu kuya na ngarlaka. Nyawa na ngarlaka na. Jiyarnana ngu jarlarlang-kula-ma ngarlaka-ma, marntaj. Ngurnayinangulu manana pakara-yirri. Nganin-ta-ma nguyinangulu ngamayi-lu nganin-ta-ma ngapulu-lu jayingana kuya.

Little Sedonyae is treated with the termite mound infusion by Violet and Leah (Photo: Felicity Meakins, 2012)

After that we turn them upside down — time for the head now. We hold them upside down, so they can inhale the smoke. We get them out of the smoke then. The mothers hold them in their laps to breastfeed.

Ngurnayinangulu kamparnana tamarra-ma tajkarra ngurnalu panana. Tamarra-ma, ngurnayinangulu nakurr karan manana karu-wu-ma. Ngurnayinangulu yuwanana yuka warlaya yuka you know kalypa. Nyawa na nakurr ngurnayinangulu kuya pirrkap manana karu-ma. Warlaya na nyawa-ngka ngurnayinangulu yuwanana yuka nyanawu kalypa. Karu-ma makin. Ngurnayinangulu kamparnana tamarra-lu na. Kamparnani ngurnayinangulu tamarra-lu, marntaj. Jangkarnik jiyarnana yalungku-ma tamarra-lu-ma. Ngu puya jangkarni karru. Mingip yanku ngu. Parntawurru ngurnayinangulu kamparnana. Ngulu lurlu karru. Ngurnayinangulu kamparnana na ngamany-ma kuya ngurnayinangulu yuwanana ngamany-ja tamarra-ma.

We cook the antbed, [put water on it] and then crush it. Then we hollow out the ground for the kids. We put the soft spinifex in [or other types of medicine like hakea]. We lay the newborn babies down and we cover them with the antbed. The antbed makes them grow up strong. It makes their bodies strong so they will be able to sit up straight and crawl. We also treat the fontanelle by putting antbed on this part of the head.

Karu kamparnup —
Treatments using termite mound

told by Biddy Wavehill

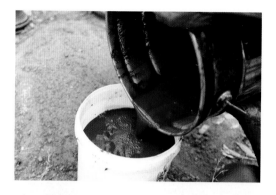

Ngayu-ma-rna malu karu-wu yapayapa-wu, newborn-baby-wu kuya. Nyamu-lu wart yanana kaarniin. Yanani kaarnirra-jirri Jinparrak-kula. Jalajala-ma medicine-ta righto. Ngurnayinangkulu karu kangani wart. Jaju-ngku-ma nyampa-ku-ma ngantipany-ju-ma-yinangkulu karrwarnani. Bush-medicine — tamarra, warlayara. Tamarra-la, murlangka kawarla-la, ngurnayinangkulu yuwanani nyila na nyampayirla. Ngurnayinangkulu karrap nyangani. Yuka yuka yeah pija. Alright put 'em karu makin. Kamparnu na tamarra-la. Might be jurlurl yuwanani one two three ngirljik you know, tamarra. Righto jumpuruk nyila-ma karu-ma. I kaan lungkarra nyampa na init. Kula karru janga nyampa. Im kill 'en germ inside.

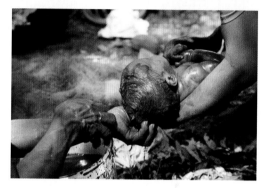

I'm going to talk about newborn babies [and what we do] when they come back from hospital. They used to come back east to old Wave Hill Station. These days there's modern medicine [but in the old days] we would bring the children back and our grannies would have some bush medicine ready for them. Some bush medicines were antbed and soft spinifex. We put them in the antbed which was in a coolamon. We used to monitor them. The stems of the spinifex [went in too]. We lay the babies down and treated them in the antbed. Then we poured the antbed mix in their mouths and they would swallow it. The babies' bodies would strengthen then. They won't cry, get sick or anything. The antbed slurry kills the germs inside the babies.

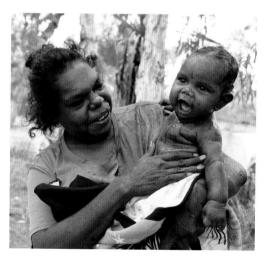

Held by her mother Christine Mick, Frankesha Djaban is treated with the antbed mix inside and out (Photo: Penny Smith, 2016)

Warlu-warla pirrkap marntaj, righto. Tamarra kankunungkarra, partaj. Right jiyarnana ngu nyila-ma tamarra-ma black one-pijik. Right nyila-ma yuka-ma kuya na tajkarra-la make 'em soft one. Put 'em langa kawarla na. Alright yalanginyi-ma warrkuj. Tajkarra-la kawarla-la-rni make 'em soft one-pijik binij. Yurtup-parla kalypak marntaj. Alright put 'em now yalangka-warla karu-ma makin. Ngirlkirri nyampa kamparnup, kankuliin ngamany. Like make 'em jiput kankuliit nyanuny ngarlaka

We make a fire, OK. The antbed goes on top then. The antbed burns until it goes black. Then you pound the soft spinifex to make it soft and you put it into a coolamon. You grind it in the coolamon until it is soft. Lay the baby in it now and slather the baby from the throat up and the fontanelle down. This makes sure the fontanelle closes.

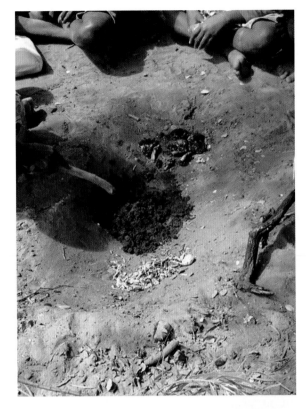

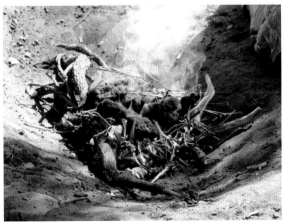

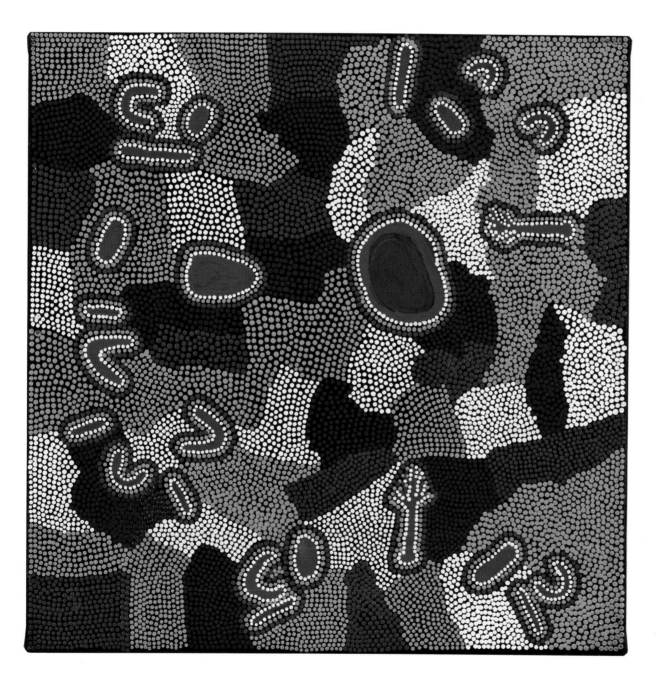

Karu Kamparnup — Treating Babies with Termite Mound
(Painting: Violet Wadrill, 2017)

Warra karu parntawurru — Looking after babies' backs

Told by Violet Wadrill

Juluj ngurnayinangkulu kangani karu-ma yapayapa-
ma. You know ngapuju ngayiny yapakayi kuya-
marraj-ma. An nyamu-lu karrinya mingip-kaji.
Lurlulurlu-waji karu kuyany-ma-rnayinangkulu til
julujuluj kangani kawarla-la-ma jangkakarni-la-ma.

We carry babies in coolamons on our hips — you
know newborn babies — and even when they have
started crawling. When they start walking, we carry
them in bigger coolamons.

Parntawurru-ma-lu yuwanani punyu, kuyangka-ma,
karu-ma. Ngurnayinangkulu ngitji karrinyani
parntawurru-wu. Ngitji ngurnayinangkulu
karrinyani karu-wu, parntawurru-wu ngaja-
lu warrngun karrinyana. That's why kawarla-la
ngurnayinangkulu kangani.

Coolamons make the children's backs straight
and strong. We get concerned about their backs
because, if we don't look after them, the children
will end up in pain. That's why we carry them in
the coolamons.

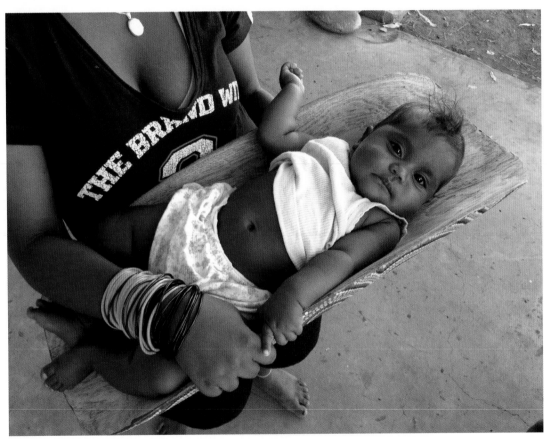

Kierita Dandy held by her mother, Jezebel Dandy (Photo: Penny Smith, 2013)

Purntunarri kamparnup — Treating older babies
told by Connie Ngarmeiye with Sarah Oscar

Ngurna mani tamarra an ngirirri. Ngurna mani karu-wu yaluwu yapakayi-wu. Ngurna kamparni fire-ngku light 'em ngurna mani. Warlu-ngku ngurna kamparni karu nyila. Ngurna kamparni lanti an nyampayirla knee. Ngurna kamparni turturl na kalu-wu. Properly way ngurna kamparni karu-ma nyila-ma parntawurru-ma an knee-kujarra. Ngurna kamparni finish. Kanya na mummy-ngku nyanuny-ju. Next time-ma im gon rarrarrajkarra everyway kalu na, dat karu.

I got some termite mound and dry hakea seeds and twigs for the baby. I lit a fire, burnt it down (put water on it and crushed it up). I slathered the baby with the warm mixture. I applied it to his hips, knees and back. I treated him with it so he could walk. Next thing you know, he was running everywhere.

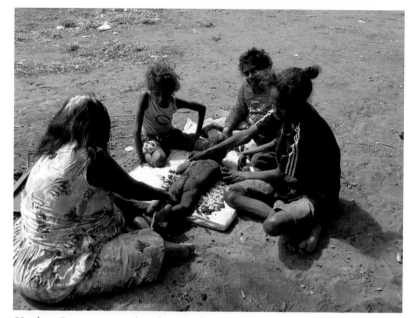

Keithan Barry is treated with antbed and hakea by Connie Ngarmeiye and his mother Lisa Smiler. Keenan Barry and Becky Peter watch on (Photo: Felicity Meakins, 2010)

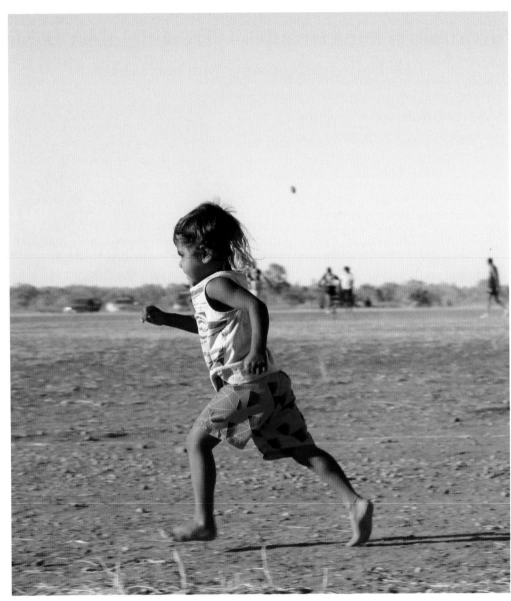

Ricco Watson tests out his strong hips and knees (Photo: Penny Smith, 2014)

Yarnanti rarraj-ku — A charm for running

sung by Dandy Danbayarri

This charm is used to sing little children's feet to help them run fast. The song comes from the Yiparrartu (Emu) Dreaming. The song should be sung to the left knee of the child. Another common use of this song in contemporary Gurindji culture is at the football field, where the legs of footballers are sung.

It begins with the declaration:

> Karu yanta!
> Rarraj yanta jirrimarna wanyjarnani nyila-ma ngumayila!
> Nyuntu-ma rarrajkarra kamparri!

> Go child!
> Run fast! Leave everyone behind!
> You run ahead!

Then the song goes:

> Karrakarrampi jinampa
> Karrakarrampi jinampa
> Karrakarrampi jinampa

> Walyawalyarri jinampa
> Walyawalyarri jinampa

> Karrakarra karrakarra karrakarrampi jinampa
> Karrakarra karrakarra karrakarra ooh

These three verses cannot be translated. It's believed they feature an ancient form of Gurindji or Mudburra, like Shakespeare or Beowulf.

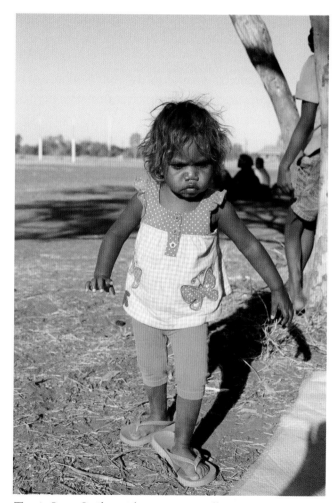

Tanzia Jerry-Smiler with grown-up walking aspirations
(Photo: Penny Smith, 2014)

Ngarrka karu-walija — Introducing children to country and ancestors
told by Violet Wadrill

Yani ngurnalu kankayit. Ngawa-ngku nguyinangulu kunyjarni malykmalyk kanyjurra yalangka, karu-walija, jangkakarni, marturtukuja an boiboi karu nyila. An jangkakarni-purrupurru wayi. Nguyinangulu kunyjarni ngawa-ngku-ma. Nyawa-ma Bilinarra kantri. Ngarinyman kantri.

When we came from upstream (from Kalkaringi to Gregory/Judbarra National Park), the traditional owner Robbie Peter sprinkled the Gurindji girls and boys with water down at the river. And the adults. He put water on their arms and heads (to introduce them to the country) because this is Bilinarra country and Ngarinyman country.

Jungkart ngurnayinangulu jayinya yalanginyi-ma, nyangka karlarra. Kamparni ngurnayinangulu jungkart-tu. Jayinya ngurnayinangulu nyampayirla marlarn ngamanpurru pakarli. Pinarrik ngurnayinangulu kamparni karu-ma nyila-ma. Ngurra-ngku murlungku im ged ngarrka nyarrulu. Ngaja-yinangulu kanginy pungku. Kamparrijang-kulu nyamu-lu-wa waninya walartarti. Kamparrijang ngumpit, kajijirri, murluwu ngurra-wu. jayinya ngurnayinangulu jungkart purrp-parni . Nguyinangulu ngarrka manku, nyamu-lu yanangku.

Next we smoked the children. We treated them with smoke from river red gum, conkerberry and paperbark leaves. We smoked them so they would get to know the country. The country will also get to know the children this way. The old people who died on this country long ago might not recognise them. Many of our ancestors were from this country. That's why we smoked all of the children — so our ancestors will know this next generation any time they come here.

Ngulu ngarrka na manangku nyawa-ma ngurra-ma, karu-ngku-ma jangkakarni na nyamu-lu karru. Yuu kuya na. Jumpurnkarra nyamu-rnayingulu kamparni. Jungkart nyamu-rnayingulu jayinya. Jungkart ngurnayinangulu jayinya pinarrik. Ngurra-ngku murlungku nguyina, ngarrka manku, nyamu-rnayinangulu kunyarni ngawa-ngku nyampa-ku. Jungkart ngurnayinangulu jayinya marlarn ngamanpurru pakarli jungkart. Jangkakarni, yapayapa, kuya.

The children will get to know this country as they get older. That's how it works when we treat them with the smoke. We smoke them to bring them into the knowledge of this country. That's also why we water them. We bathe the adults and kids alike in the smoke from river red gum, conkerberry and paperbark.

Centipede ngurramala ngu. Karrinya murlangka ngu tanjarri nyantu-ma Sanford-ta. Well pina ngurla murlarniny ngurra-wu na. Yani yawarta-lu jalajalngak. Kangani murlangkurra-ma-lu pinarrik. Robbie im know, nyawa ngurra nyanany. Ngamayi kantri, jawiji kantri. Im Bilinarra karu, nyantu-ma, ngamayi nyamu-rla jawiji-purrupurru Ngarinyman-purru Bilinarra.

Robbie Peter 'Centipede' is the traditional owner. He grew up at Mt Sanford Station. So he knows all about this country. He used to ride this country on a horse. The old people used to take him here so he could learn. This is why Robbie knows his country. It's his mother's and maternal grandfather's country. He's a Bilinarra child through his mother and maternal grandfather who were Ngarinyman and Bilinarra.

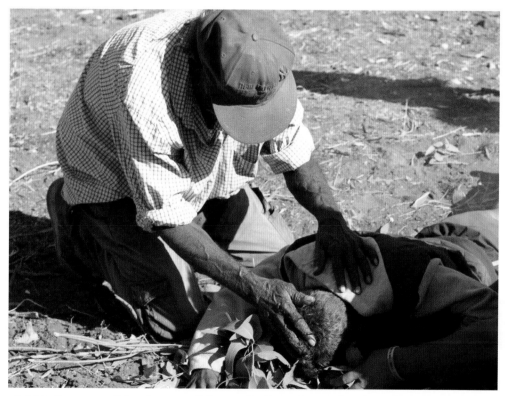

Robbie Peter, a traditional owner of Gregory/Judbarra National Park smokes Keithan Barry
at Paperbark Yard to introduce the country and ancestral traditional owners to him.
The smoke also helps settle down children. (Photo: Penny Smith, 2018)

Manyanyi and marlarn — Bush vicks and river red gum

told by Biddy Wavehill

Jangkarni-piya na purntunarri, im kamat skin na. Nyila-ma manyanyi, marlarn, taruk. Tarukap-kula marntaj, righto jumpurn ngaja janga karrinyana. Nomo ngajik janga. Like jumpurn you know kuyangku ngarlaka-ngurlung minti-ngurlung like, finish.

Now the baby's a bit bigger — big enough to crawl. Now it's time to smoke her with bush vicks and river red gum to prevent her from getting sick. She'll stay well this way. She's smoked from head to toe.

Bush Vicks: *Blumea, Streptoglossa, Pterocaulon spp.*
River Red Gum: *Eucalyptus camaldulensis*

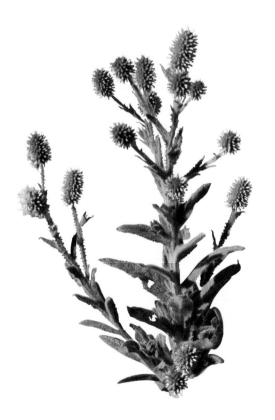

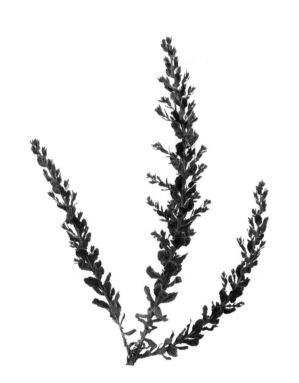

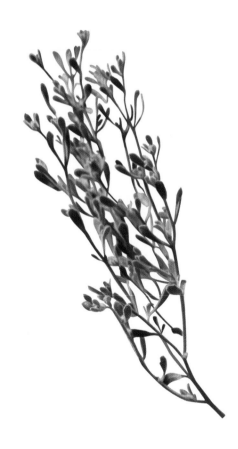

Yarnanti kulykulya-wu — A charm for colds

sung by Dandy Danbayarri

This charm is used to sing away the symptoms of a cold:

Kulykulya murrunpungku murrunpungku
Kulykulya murrunpungku murrunpungku
Kulykulya murrunpungku murrunpungku
Karlajirri murrunpungu
Karlajirri murrunpungu

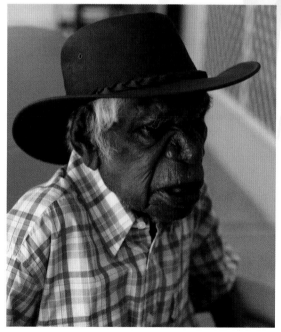

Dandy Danbayarri (Photo: Penny Smith, 2016)

Punyukkaji kulykulya-wu — Cures for colds

told by Kitty Mintawurr and Biddy Wavehill
with Violet Wadrill

Nyawa marlarn, karu-walija-ma tarukap ngurnayinangulu murlangka na medicine-ta tarukap. Jangkakarni too. Ngurnalu waninyana nyamu-rnalu kulyakap karrinyana. Ngurnalu yuwanana bakit-ta boil 'em. Ngurnalu gone outside-jirri. Coolbalak karrinyana nyantu-rni. Taruk na ngurnalu yuwanana. Ngapuk-ma marlarn-parni, tarukap-ma.

The leaves of river red gums also make a good medicinal wash. We wash the kids in it — adults too. We bathe in it when we have a cough. We put it in a bucket and boil it. Then we take it off [the fire] and wait until the medicinal wash cools down. We bathe in it then. You can really smell it when you bathe in it.

Nyawa-ma-rnalu manana manyanyi tarukap-ku nyamu-lu karrinyana karu-walija ichy. An nyamu-lu karrinyana kulykulya-yawung ngurnalu manana nyawa na ngunayinangkulu tarukap yuwanana murlungku, nyawa manyanyi-ma.

We also get bush vicks to wash the kids when they are itching. Or if they are congested, we also pick bush vicks and bathe them in it.

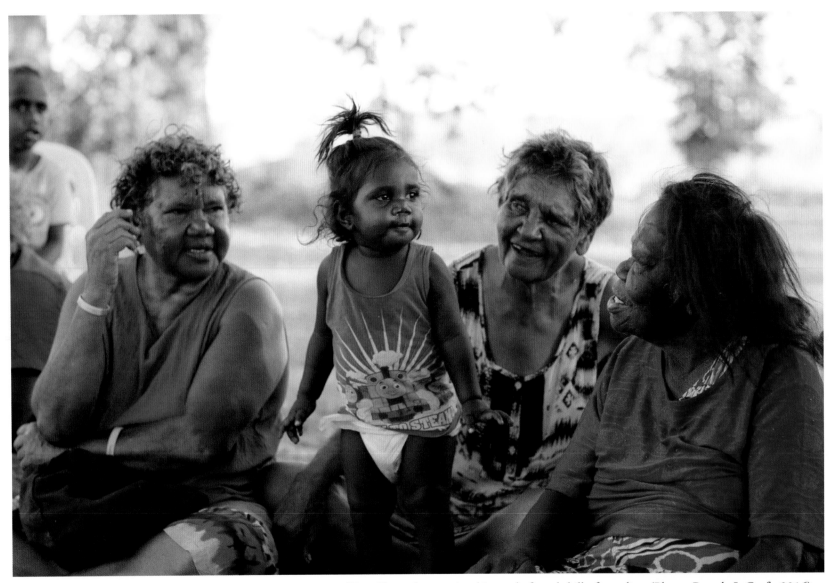

Kathy Wardill, Pauline Ryan and Connie Ngarmeiye encourage Troy Alec as he practises his newly found skill of standing (Photo: Brenda L Croft, 2016)

Yirrijkaji, wariyili and partiki —
Dodonaea polyzyga, Senna spp., Terminalia arostrata
told by Violet Wadrill and Biddy Wavehill

Jangkakarni-wu-purrupurru ngurnayinangulu kamparnana murluny-jawung-kulu-ma yirrijkaji-yawung-kulu. Nyawa-ma yirrijkaji-ma kamparnup marntara-yawung-ku nyampa-wu, kulykulya-wu, ngarlaka-wu wankaj-ku kuyawu karu-purrupurru nyamu-lu-wa karrinyana ngajkula-yawung-ku jumpurn ngurnayinangulu kamparnana nyawa-yawung-kulu.

We also smoke people with *yirrijkaji* by putting the leaves on warm coals until it smokes. We use it for people with head sores, congestion or a headache. We also smoke kids with this kind of medicine when they have diarrhoea.

Nyila na wariyili im punyu nyila-ma. Boil 'em-kula-ma im kuyany winkilying. Karu janga ngurnayinangulu yuwanana mantara-yawung. Nyamu-lu karrinyana ngarlaka-la maru-ngka nyampa-ka. Marntara yaluny-jawung-kulu-ma, punyu tarukap-ku-ma. Bush-medicine nyila-ma wariyili-ma.

The wariyili tree also has medicinal properties. When you boil it, the water goes red. We bathe children with it when they have skin sores or scabies on their heads or bottoms or anywhere. This type of plant is good for treating sores. It is a type of bush medicine.

Partiki nyawa, nyila jintapa-kari-ma, janga-yawung-ku-ma karlapa-wu-purrupurru. Karlapa-ma nyamu-lu karrinyana, ngurnayinangulu kamparnana kuyangku-ma. Wilyjirrij nyawa ngurla-nyanta yanana, nyila-ma karlapa-ma. Jik ngurla yanana jangkarni-ma. Kangarnta ngurnalu tal panana nyila-ma wurrkal-ma. Marntara-wu nyampa-wu karlapa-wu, janga-yawung-ku kuyany-ma im punyu.

The bark from a young nut tree is another one which can be used [to treat] kids with skins sores, scabies or boils. If they have boils, we bathe them and the pus comes out. A lot can come out. We call this green stuff the 'mouth' of the boil.

Nganany karu-wu — Warnings for children

told by Violet Wadrill

Jikirrij — Willie-wagtail

"Nyamu-n-nga parru tampang ngamayi-ma ngu tampang karru!" kuya. Kuya-waji na nyawa-ma. Marnani ngulu-rla, nyawa-wu-ma jikirrij-ku-ma. "Nomo parra, kuya, ngaja ngamayi ngaji ngaja-ngku-rla tampang karru!"

"Your mother will die if you kill a willy-wagtail!" That's what they used to say about the willy-wagtail. "Don't kill it or your mother and father might die!"

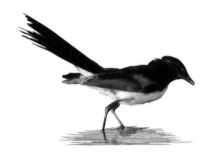

Jikirrij (Willy-wagtail, *Rhipidura leucophrys*) (Photo: Bob Gosford)

Wirnangpurru — Kangaroo

Nyanawu pilyily yapakayi majul-la nyamu kangana puul-la walyak. Pilyily-ma. Pilyily nyila wirnangpurru. Kula-n manku patpat. Nyamu yanana purlp yapakayi pilyily, karu-ngku yalangku kula manku. Ngaja karrinyana tingarri-kujarra wankaj. Purlppurlpkarra-la-ma. Nyila-ma wirnangpurru nyamu-n manana yapakayi-ma pilyily, kula manku pat-ma karu-ngku-ma, lawara, ngaja karrinyana tingarri wankaj. Kuya na nguyinangulu marnani-ma, kirri-ma kamparrijang. Nomo manku-rla pat nyila, wirnangpurru yapawurru, pilyily ngaja nyampayirla yuwanana wankajirrik manana tingarri-ma. Marntaj.

You know the hairless joey that is still in its mother's pouch. The one that's just been born. Well children shouldn't touch that one. Even when it is big enough to hop a little way from its mother, don't let a child get it either. The child's knees will be affected and they will end up limping. That's what the women told us in the old days. You shouldn't touch young baby kangaroos because it's bad for babies' knees. That's what they reckoned.

Jarrakap — Learning to talk

Children the world over go through different stages when they are learning to talk, from babbling to a one-word stage to using multiple words. Gurindji children are no different, but they often learn some *takataka* (sign language) before acquiring speech. *Takataka* is used throughout the community to supplement speech in situations where someone is out of earshot, for example in a car, or with deaf members of the community. Sometimes children are slow to learn language or cannot articulate words clearly, a condition called *karrjan* ('double tongue'). In some cases, adults intervene to speed up their progress. The eggs of a bird called a *panaka* can be collected and smeared on children's tongues, or an adult will warm her thumb and index finger over a fire and pull a child's tongue out. These techniques are said to shock children into speaking. If a child continues muteness into adulthood, they are referred to as *amama*.

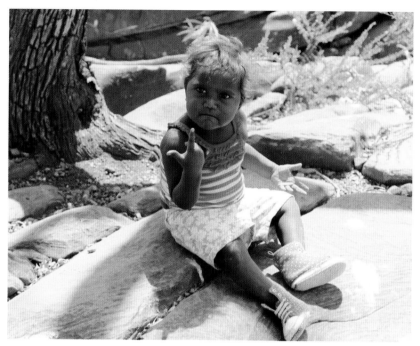

Meiye Roy signs "What's up?" to her mother (Photo: Penny Smith, 2015)

Janyarrp — Baby talk

In some cultures, adults talk to young children in *janyarrp* (baby talk) which they believe helps their learning. Gurindji adults use *janyarrp* with their young children. *Janyarrp* consists of some words which are totally different from adult words. For example *kakkak* is the baby talk word for something dangerous or yucky, whereas the normal Gurindji words are *kuliyan* or *wankaj*. Sometimes in *janyarrp*, the adult Gurindji word is used, but some sounds are dropped. The *janyarrp* word for 'milk' is *apu* which drops sounds at the beginning and end of the adult word *ngapulu*. In other *janyarrp*, sounds are changed, for example *kungulu* becomes *kukulu*. The cutest form of *janyarrp* is when adults change 't' to 'j' and 'n' to 'ny', for example *karnti* 'tree' is pronounced *kanyji*. On the next page are some more examples of *janyarrp*.

Special baby talk words

English	Gurindji	Janyarrp
food	tanku	nyanya
dangerous or yucky	kuliyan, wankaj	kakkak
poo	kura	kaka
sore	janga	juu

Palatalisations

English	Gurindji	Janyarrp
old man	marluka	malyuka
milk, breast	ngapulu	ngapulyu
tree, branch	karnti	kanyji
climb	partaj	pajaj

Sounds dropped

English	Gurindji	Janyarrp
milk	ngapulu	apu, papu and apulu
grandmother	ngapuju	apuju
water	ngawa	awa
little	yapakayi	apakayi

Sounds changed

English	Gurindji	Janyarrp
head	ngarlaka	warlaka
cry	lungkarra	lungkaya
bird	jurlaka	kurlaka
blood	kungulu	kukulu

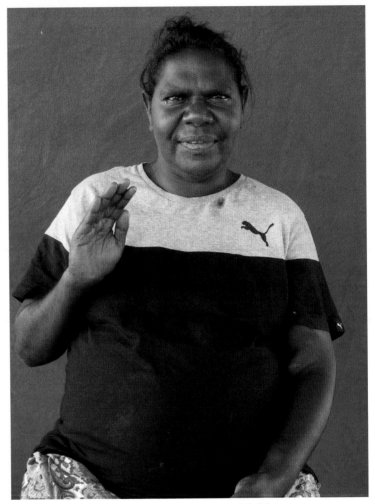

Cedrina Algy demonstrates the sign for *karu* (child)
(Photo: Jennifer Green, 2017)

Jaru karu-wu — Words for babies

Ngarturr — pregnant woman

Ngamayi — mother

Ngamarlang — mother and child

Purirripurirri — camp for a woman who has just had a baby

Nganymanta — newborn baby, literally 'in a cradle'

Parlarra — baby born with no hair

Yapakaru — tiny baby

Milarntakaru — baby still in a coolamon

Ngapuluwaji — breastfeeding baby

Tamparrpkaji — baby who lies on its tummy but can hold her head up to look around

Wumpulungkaji — baby who can roll

Lurluwaji — baby who can sit up

Purntunarri, mingipkaji — baby who can crawl

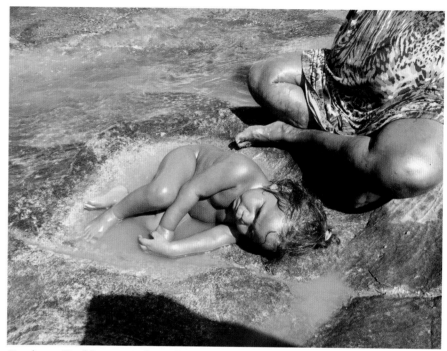

Reeshawn Dodd practises his rolling in the cool at Lawi
(Photo: Penny Smith, 2016)

Kaluwaji — toddler

Yuwupkaji — baby who can babble

Jarrakapkaji — talking stage

Janyarrp — baby talk

Lungkarrapkaji, wajiwurru — cry baby

Jajarra — child who no longer receives milk from their mother because she is expecting another child

Pulkunga — eldest child

Pulkunga jarrara — second child, literally – accompanying the eldest

Kamurrkamurr — middle child

Kurtpu jarrara — youngest child, literally – accompanying the lower leg

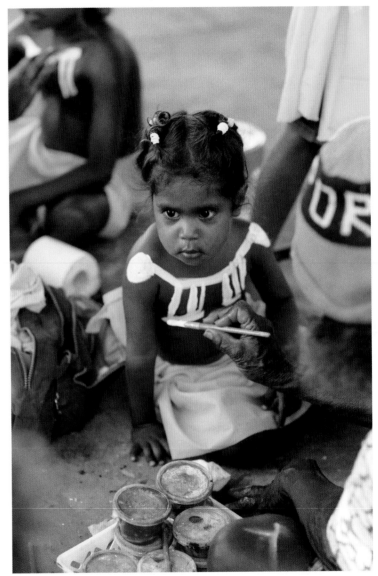

Kierita Dandy is painted up by Violet Wadrill for dancing
(Photo: Brenda L Croft, 2016)

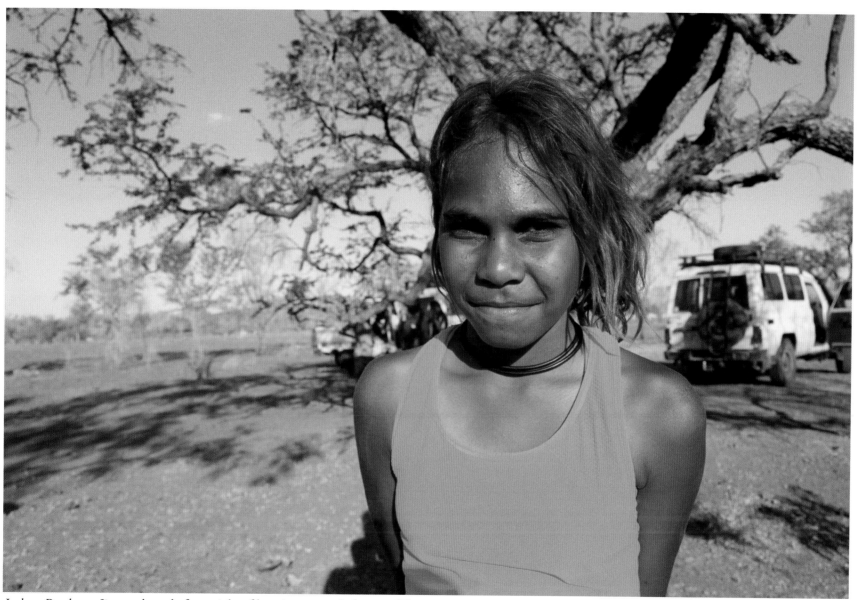

Jaylene Barclay at Jinparrak ready for a night of learning women's dancing (Photo: Penny Smith, 2016)

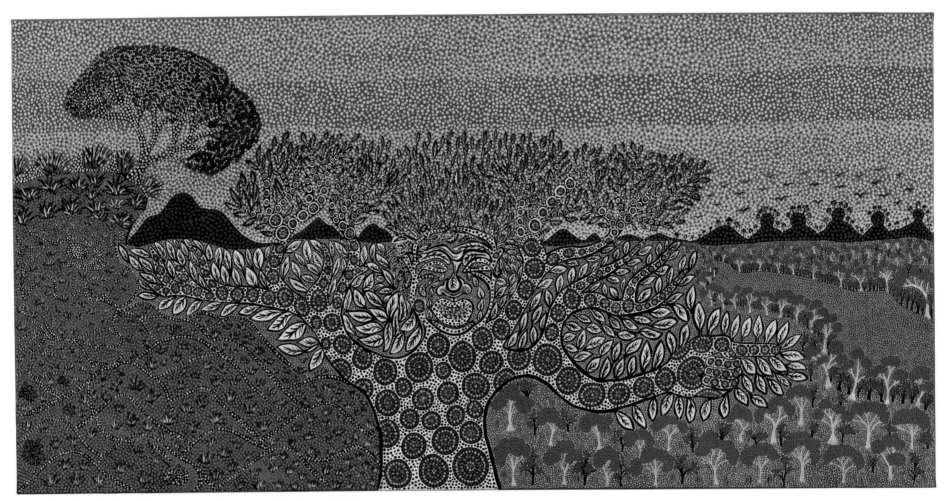

Jampurra — The Cry Baby (Painting: Desmarie Morrison, 2017)

Karu yurrk

Children's stories

Introduction

Like Grimm's Fairy Tales, many children's stories have grisly conclusions. Either children befall terrible fates or children are the perpetrators of dreadful acts of violence. It seems that children the world over are entertained by other people meeting horrible ends! For example, in *Jajurlang*, the grandson kills his grandmother when she consistently refuses to give him water after unsuccessful hunting trips. In *Ngarlking Karu*, the son surreptitiously eats his parents' food. One night they abandon him while he sleeps and he later wreaks his revenge by creating a drought, ultimately killing his parents.

The stories are told by Violet Wadrill, a highly respected Gurindji storyteller. Violet tells the stories in Gurindji, but in one of the stories, *Jajurlang*, the characters talk in Jaru a language spoken west of Gurindji country. Ena Oscar also recalls her mother telling a version of the story in

Some of the artists, Violet Wadrill, Ena Oscar, Rosemary Johnston and Narelle Morris listen to Violet's stories played by Felicity Meakins to get inspiration for their paintings (Photo: Penny Smith, 2017)

Mudburra when she was a child. Mudburra country is located east of Gurindji country. The fact that these stories can be told in different languages with no reference to landmarks and no place names shows their universality as children's stories. They are not owned by any family nor are they associated with specific country. The stories are freely told to children across the region in different ways and with local flavours. The use of multiple languages in these stories also shows Violet's mastery of languages.

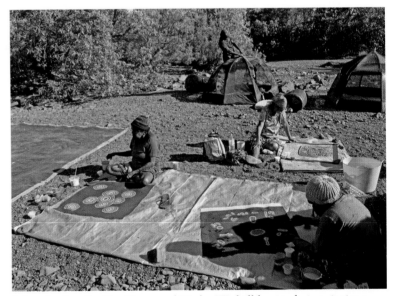

Mary Smiler, Pauline Ryan and Violet Wadrill begin their paintings (Photo: Penny Smith, 2017)

The artworks associated with the stories (and throughout this book) were created during a Karungkarni Arts camp run in July 2017 and supported by the Murnkurrumurnkurru Central Land Council ranger group. Participating artists were Violet Wadrill, Ena Oscar, Rosemary Johnson, Sarah Oscar, Mary Smiler, Narelle Morris, Pauline Ryan and Tara Long. They listened to the stories on the first evening of the camp to get inspiration for their paintings. Violet was present, allowing artists to discuss the details of the stories with her. For the next two days the artists completed their works. The location of the camp was Warrijkuny (Sambo Rockhole) on the Victoria River, 50 km from Kalkaringi, which is Topsy Dodd Ngarnjal's country. Topsy gave her permission for the group to camp on her country and for Violet to tell the *Warrija Kirrawa* story associated with the rockhole. Some of the artists also decided to depict this story in their paintings. One of Violet's other stories, *Jampurra*, describes country on the eastern side of Limbunya Station (Malngin country located 100 km west of Kalkaringi). The *Luma Kurrupartu* story, a Dreaming story which comes from the same area, is also included in this chapter. Like many of these stories, it shares important information about country.

– **Felicity Meakins**

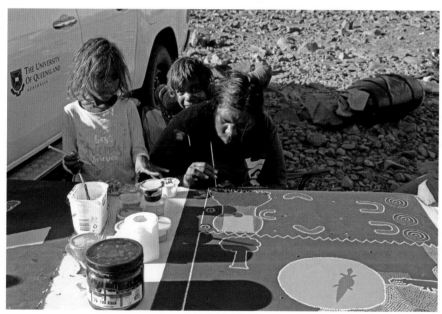

Narelle Morris painting with her children Dylena and Reuben
(Photo: Penny Smith, 2017)

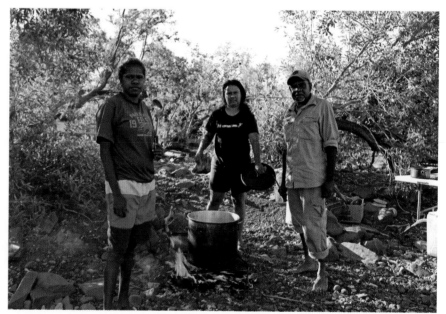

Murnkurrumurnkurru Central Land Council rangers Helma Bernard, Ursula Chubb
and Philip Jimmy cook for the artists (Photo: Penny Smith, 2017)

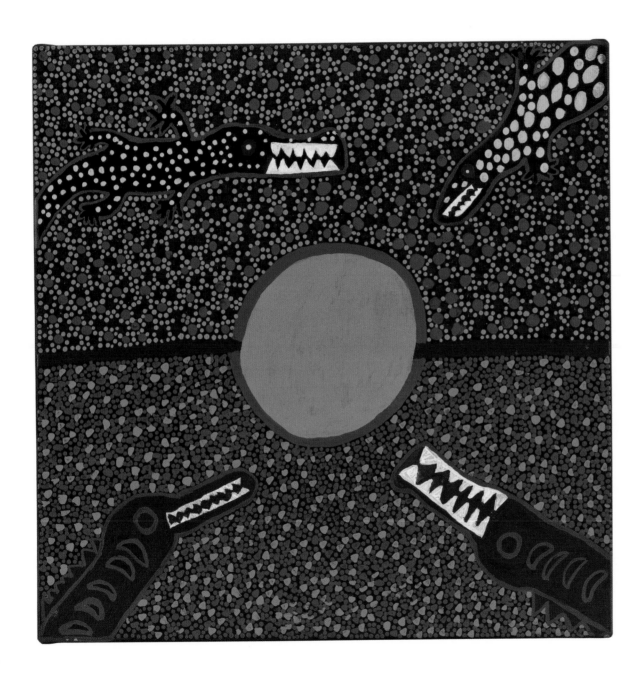

Warrija Kirrawa — The Crocodile and Goanna
(Painting: Sarah Oscar, 2017)

"Yeah nyangka-yi-rla." Yani na nganta warrij, Kirrawa-ma. Yani warrij nyila-ma Kirrawa-ma nganta, warlakap na ngurla nyangani. Martiya-wu ngurla nyangani pirijpirij-kari pirijpirij-kari karnti you know karnti martiya-waji. Nyila na.

Nganta-rla mani puntanup-parla, nyampayirla-lu-ma, Kirrawa-ngku-ma. Puntanup ngurla mani nyampayirla-ma martiya-ma marntaj. Kangani na ngurla. Kirrawa-lu-ma wart na ngurla kangani. "Nyampa nganta-rnangku kangana ngayu! Punyu ngurnangku kangana, majka ngurnangku-rla. Kawayi na!"

Nyila-ma Warrija-ma-rla yani na, jarlapalkarra jarlapal kuya. Warrija-ma jarlapal na karrinyana. Ngurla marni na Kirrawa-ma, "Ngurnangku-rla majka yuwarru nyawa-ja, martiya-ma-kata." Ngurla yuwani palnyangpalnyang na nyila-ma martiya-ma nyanuny-ja-ma, kuyarniny-side-ta-ma, yaluwu-ma nyampa-warla-ma Warrija-wu-ma. Ngurla yuwani palnyangpalnyang Kirrawa-lu-ma marntaj.

"Well ngali yanku-rli, ngawa-ngkurra na! Ngurnangku marlu-warluk-parni. Nyamu-rna-nga ngayu ngajik-parni yanku kanyjurra," ngurla marni Warrija-ma. "Nyamu-rna-nga ngayu ngajik-parni tarap yanku, kuyangka-ma nyuntu-ma yanta kaja-ngkurra na. Kaja-ngka na karra. Nomo ngawa-ngkurra yanta wart-kari," ngurla marni nyila-ma Warrija-ma. "Ngayu-ma-rna-nga yanku ngawa-ngkurra-ma."

"Yeah you look for something for me." Goanna must have left then. He headed off, searching for something. He was looking for bush gum — or a *pirijpirij* tree, you know the trees that bush gum comes from. That one now.

Goanna collected the bush gum. He kept collecting the gum. Then Goanna took it back for him. "Look! I'm bringing you something. I'm bringing you something good to give a go. Come here!"

Crocodile went to him then, slithering along on his belly. Crocodiles have their bellies close to the ground! Goanna said to him, "I'll try and put the bush gum on you." He stuck the gum all along Crocodile's back and tail. Goanna stuck it all over him until there was none left.

"Hey let's go into the water now! First, I want to tell you something though. If I go underwater, it might be for a while," Crocodile said to him, "If I dive under, it might be forever. So you should go to the land and stay there. You shouldn't come back to the water again," Crocodile explained to him. "Me, well I'm entering the water now."

Jirrpu wanku na ngajik-parni na nyila-ma, kanyjurra-ma ngawa-ngka-ma. "Nyamu-n-nga nyampa-wu yaluwu jarrakap-ku, kula-rna yanku wart-kari." Yani ngu kanyjurra-ma, Warrija-ma jirrpu-ma waninya ngawa-ngka-ma. Ngajik-parni tarap waninya.

Ngurla nyangani Kirrawa-lu-ma nganta karrap. "Wanyji yanana jaliji ngayiny. Wanyji wart yanana. Lawara. Ah nyila-ma nyamu-yi marni. Ngurna yanku kaja-ngkurra ngayu-ma ngajik-parni. Kaja-ngka karru-rna-nga. Nyila-ma yani ngawa-ngkurra-ma ngajik-parni na. Ngawa jirrpu na waninya. Marntaj.

And so he was going to dive down into the water forever. "Even if you come back to tell me a story or some news, I won't come back again," said Crocodile. Down Crocodile went, diving deep underwater. He dived down never to be seen again.

Goanna would watch for him. "Where did my friend go? Will he come back? I guess not. That is what he said to me. Well I guess I'll have to live on land permanently. I might live on land since Crocodile went into the water for good." That's the end of the story!

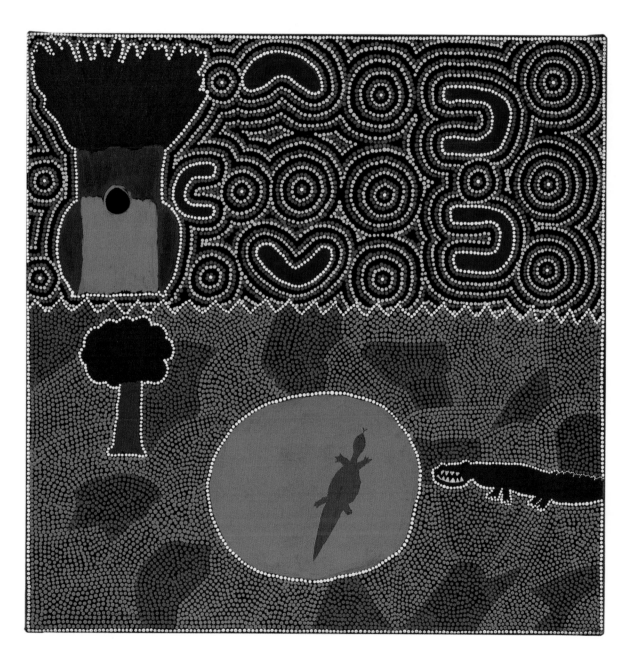

Warrija Kirrawa — The Crocodile and Goanna
(Painting: Narelle Morris, 2017)

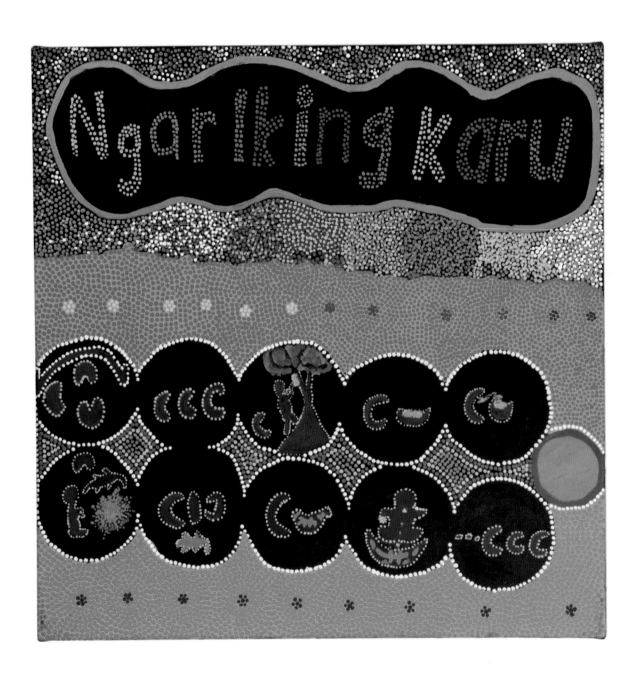

Ngarlking Karu — The Greedy Boy
(Painting: Sarah Oscar, 2017)

Ngarlking karu — The greedy child

told by Violet Wadrill Nanaku to Marie Japan Nangari

Karu-ma yala-ma nganta yanani ngu ngaji-wu nga nga. Tuwa nganta-rla yanani ngaji-wu-ma. Ngantuku-rla yuwarru, jalak ngamayi-wu ngarlu. "Ngaji," kuya. Nyila-ma nganta-rla jayingana, "Kutirni kutirni liwart ngurnangku-rla yuwarru nyawa, parnngirri-la. Nganta ngaji nyantu-ma yuwanani parnngirri-la-ma nyila-ma ngarlu-ma, kuya.

"Kanku ngurna-rla ngamayi-wu na." Kangani nganta kamparra-rni ngarnani nganta init Nangari. Kamparra-rni, ngarnani ngu binij. Dat ngarlu, middle-la-rni kamurra-la.

"I'll take it to Mum now." He took it but stopped halfway and ate it. He ate the whole lot! He gobbled down all of the honey halfway there.

Yanani ngurla ngamayi-wu jik. Kurrijkarra ngamayi-lu-ma nganta. Put 'em kawarla-la-ma wayita-ma. Wayita-walija-ma nganta put 'em kawarla-la-ma. Yangunungku-nganyjuk ngamayi-lu-ma im take 'em julujuluj, punkulung-kula kuyany-ja jangkarni-la nganta.

Then he went up to his mother. She was digging up some pencil yams and putting them in a coolamon. She put lots of yams in her coolamon. Then she hauled up her yams and bush potatoes on her hip.

There was a child who went up to his father. He approached his father who wanted him to deliver some honey to his mother. "Hi Dad!" he said. His father gave him something saying, "Wait up, I'll wrap you something in paperbark to give to your mother." So his father put some honey in some paperbark for him.

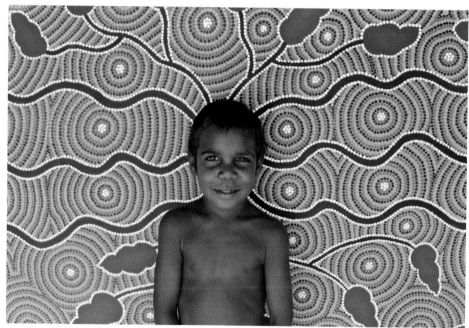

Reuben Miller with a bush potato painting created by his father Dylan Miller (Photo: Penny Smith, 2014)

"Ngama. Ngunkurla ngaji-wu, jalak yuwarru, wayita, an nyampayirla kamara, yangunungku?" Jayingani nganta-rla ngamayi-lu-ma, jiwirri you know cooked one wayita. "Kangka-rla na. Kangka-rla. Ngaji-wu kangka-rla.

Kangani nganta nyila-ma wayita-ma kamparnu-nginyi-ma. Kamurra-la-rni jaartkarra. Middle-la imin already finish 'em kuyangku. Jaartkarra tanku.

Im gu langa im na ngaji-wu nyanuny-ku. "Nganta-nkurla yuwarru ngamayi-wu? Kirrawa might be yapayapa you know kirrawa nyampayirla." Kaja-ngka nyamu-rla panani nyanawu nyampayirla-purrupurru, ngarranginy-purrupurru. Ngarranginy-purrupurru nyamu-lu panana kaja-ngka you know marlurluka-lu. An ngulu kangani kuya na wirriji-la kuya.

Kamparnup-nginyi-ma nyila-ma, im jalak langa im na. "Ngaji ngunkurla kirrawa yujuk parru ngamanti-wu, ngamayi-wu. Im gibit im na. Might be im take 'em nyampayirla-la you know, pakarli-la lajap. Nyila kurnka im take 'em murlangka jijpart wirriji-la. Kangani na ngurla, nyila-ma kirrawa-ma. Might be yapayapa you know kuyakijak good size that one.

Kangani ngurla darrei kamurra im jidan. Im pilap la im nganta ngaji-wu-ma. "Ah yikili na!" Yalangka-rni ngarnana jaartkarra purrp. Im gu tanku na nganta, ngamayi-wu na. Kuya-rni nganta.

"Mum! Do you want to send some yams and potatoes to Dad?" So his mother gave him some cooked bush yams. "Take them to him now. Take it to your father."

So he took the bush yams after they were cooked. But he ate them halfway back. He finished them off halfway back just like that. He ate until he was full.

He went up to his father then. "Do you want to send some tucker for Mum? Maybe a small goanna or something?" So his father killed a frill-necked lizard he'd found for her in the bush. (Men used to hunt frill-necked lizards in the old days. They used to carry them tied with hair string around their waists with the heads hanging down).

After cooking the lizard, he got it ready to send it to his wife. "Dad — do you want me to deliver it to Mum now?" So he gave it to him. Maybe he took it tied up in some paperbark on his shoulder. Or maybe he took the cooked meat tucked in his hair belt held on with hair string. Anyway he set off, apparently taking the goanna to her. Maybe it was as big as this — a good size.

The boy started taking it to her, but stopped halfway. He looked back over his shoulder for his father. "Ah it's OK — he's a long way off!" Right there, he gobbled it all up. Then he went to his mother with a full belly. He really behaved like this!

Tubala bin tapu mijelp night time na. Ngijingka-la-ma mum-kula-ma. Tubala bin put 'em nyawa na nganta makin. Nyawa-ngka nganta fire nyawa-ngka-ma fire. Nyawa ngamayi, nyawa karu, nyawa ngaji-nyan. Olabat makin na. Ngu nganta purrngiyip na dat karu, tirrirnkarra.

"Walima-ngku kangana ngayi nyamu-rnangku yujuk panani, kirrawa?" "Lawara!" Imin purrp majurru-rni kamurra-rni. An im ask 'em ngumparna nyanuny. "Nyununy-ja wayita nyamu-rnangku yujuk panani, yangunungku?" "Lawara!" Ngarnani ngu kamurra-la-rni kamurra-la-rni, purrp jaartkarra kuya. Kamurra-la-rni. "Wartayi! Wanyjarru-rli kuyany ngarlking-ma," ngurla-rla marni. "Wanyjarru-rli!"

Ngaji-nyan bin ged 'em tamarra imin put 'em this way. Termite you know kuyarniny imin put 'em langa im. Nyawa ngurla yani ngamayi-lu jintapa-kari ngurla-rla yuwani. Nyawa-warla karu-ma makin.

Wanyjarni na nguwula, night time-parni. Wanyjarni nguwula warrij na nguwula yani. Kula-wula-rla karrinya luyurr majul-ma yaluwu-ma karu-wu-ma. Wanyjarni nguwula tumaji ngarlking. Ngarnani purrpkarra kamurrkamurra-la-rni. Tanku-ma ngarnani purrpkarra. Wanyjarni nguwula.

His parents went to bed hungry that night. The two of them put their son to sleep between them. Then they made a fire on either side of them. Here was the mother, the boy and the father. They all went to sleep then. The child snored and farted away.

"Did you get the goanna meat I sent you?" said the father. "No," replied the mother. (The boy had finished it all halfway of course!) And she asked her husband, "Did you get the bush yams and potatoes I sent?" "No!" (Again the child had eaten it all halfway back!) "Goodness me! Let's leave this greedy boy!" they said to each other. "Let's abandon him!"

His father got some heated termite mound and put it on either side of the boy (to trick him into thinking he was sleeping between warm bodies). The mother went and got another piece to put on either side of him. The boy slept on.

So his parents left him in the middle of the night. They just left him there. They didn't feel bad for the boy. They left him because he was greedy. He had been finishing all of the food halfway back. He would eat all of the tucker. So the two of them left him.

Kaputkaput na, tuliny na yani. "Ngamayi wanyjika-rla ngamayi ngamayi wanyjika-rla? Ngaji?" kuya. Lawara nganta-wuliny kuyangku-ma nyanya kuyangku-ma najing. "Nguyiwula wanyjarni," yurrk na ngurla imin track 'em jamana-la tubala yurrk. Kuya-rni kuya-rni ngurla yani kuya. Yani yangkarra-la-ma nyila-ma karu-ma nganta. "Wanyjika yani wanyjika," singing out-karra. "Ngamanti ngaji?" kuya. Lawara. Yikili nguwula wanyjarni.

Yani na nyila-ma karu-ma nganta. Yani nyila-ma karu-ma, jangkarni na karrinya. Nyantu-warij-ja-rni jangkarni. Yani nganta jangkarni-ma, well. Nyampayirla na jangkarni na karrinya. Kaja-ngka-rni, yani, ngawa na nganta mani init. Ngawa imin fill 'em up la bottle tree init. Clever one na nganta karru nyila-ma, karu-ma. Ngapaku-ma nganta everywhere-nginyi-ma. Jangkarni la big bottle tree. Yalangka na yuwani walyalyak ngawa-ma. Mani pull 'em ngawa-ma wanyjikijak kuyanginyi-ma, jintaku-la yuwani. Ngapuku-ma.

Kurrupartu na yinkarni init Nangari. This story ngungantipangulu marnani jarrakap ngantipanguny. Im Dreamtime na like Puwarraj you know. Yuwanani ngulu. Yinkarnani kurrupartu na marntaj. Mirta nyampa yinkarnani binij. Karrwarnani liwart na. Yalangka-ma bottle tree-ngka-ma liwart karrwarnani.

Early in the morning the boy got up. "Mum, where are you? Dad?" He looked around for the two of them, but couldn't see them. "They've abandoned me!?" So he tracked them by foot. That's how he went after them. The child followed them. "Where have you gone, where are you?" he called out. "Mum, Dad?" he called. But it was all in vain. They'd left him a long way behind.

The child walked on. He kept travelling until he was grown up. He grew up on his own. As an adult, he kept travelling. Well he was an adult now. Right through the bush he kept going, and he collected water from everywhere. He filled up a bottle tree with the water. The boy had become a cleverman. He drew water from everywhere. It was a big bottle tree. He put all of the water inside the tree. This part of the story is about this water.

Then he made a boomerang, didn't he Marie? This is a story that they used to tell us. It's a Dreamtime story. People used to tell this story before. He shaped some wood into a boomerang until it was finished. Then he made a shield and a few other things. He held them and waited by the bottle tree.

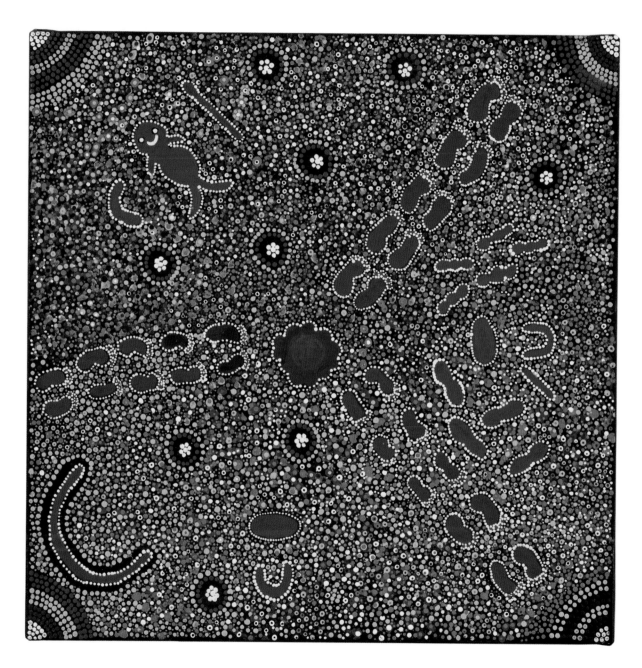

Ngarlking Karu — The Greedy Boy
(Painting: Rosemary Johnson, 2017)

Everywhere nganta everywhere ngulu-ma nyangani, "That way that way ngawa-ma! Pilyipkarra-ma karrinyana, ngapungapuku-la ngurra-ngka-ma," ngulu marnani. Nyila pilyipkarra-ma ngawa-ma karrinyana kuya. Day and night nganta they bin after 'em that ngawa. Pinka-ma everywhere-ma karrinya no nguku. Only nguku-ma yalangka-rni jintaku-la. Tumaji pull 'em mani karu-ngku yalungku-ma jintaku-yirri yuwani bottle tree-ngkurra. Yalangkawu. Tirrip-parni kalu-ma-lu yanani-ma karu-ma, marlurluka-ma, kajijirri-ma jangkakarni-ma.

Kuyangku nganta, ngamayi ngaji-ma-wula nyanya. Tuwa na ngulu yani yalangkawu ngurra-ngkawu. Kuya-ma nganta-lu karrap-ma nyanya, dat karu na wen tubala bin leave 'em im. Kuya-ma nganta-wula-rla nganta-ma ngamayi-ma ngaji-ma rarraj-ma. Kurrupartu jeya na. Wart-pari rarraj nganta-wula yanana.

"Nomo ngarrka manta-yiwula nyamu-yinpula warlaku-marraj-ma wanyjarni! Kula-rnangkula ngawa-ma yuwarru," kuya. "Nguyinpula makin-ta wanyjarni. Kula-rnangku-rla jayingku ngawa-ma."

Kuya manta-wula-rla yanani you know wijkuk kuya. Najing kurrupartu-lu-rni wart nguwuliny yanani. Panani nguwuliny kurrupartu-yawung-kulu. Kuya-rni nganta well kirri na ngurla jayinya. "Hey lamparra-marnany-ju-ma-ngku jayinya kujarra kirri kujarra nyununy.

Everyone everywhere was looking around saying "That way, that way, there's the water! Lightning is striking in that area," they said. Lightning flashed everywhere. Day and night they had been looking for water. All of the rivers were dry. There was only water in that one place because the boy had drawn it from everywhere and put it all in that one bottle tree. They had been walking all through the night (looking for water) — all of the children, men, women and adults.

Then the mother and father saw their boy. They came up close to his camp. They stared at the child who they'd just up and left. They ran up to him. But he was brandishing a boomerang! So they ran back again.

"Don't think you can claim to know me after you left me like a dog! I'm not going to give you two any water," he said. "You abandoned me while I was sleeping. So I'm not going to give you any water!"

They approached him anyway. But he threw a boomerang at them and they scuttled back. The boomerang hit them. So they decided to give him some wives. "Hey your father-in-law will give you two women!"

Ngapulu-la-ma nyawa nganta-wula. Nyampayirla-yawung-paju marrkinti-yawung. Kamparrijang-ma-lu yanani. Kuyarniny-ja ngirlkirri-la ngulu kangani kuya-marraj na, nyamu-lu yuwanani you know seed init. Kirri-ngku, nyampayirla-la wirriji-la tingkirt yuwanani kuyany-ma. Nyawa-kijak marrkanti-yawung.

"Yanta-wula-rla! Ngungalang ngawa yuwarru let 'em go." Kirri-kujarra-ma parnmarra-kujarra, ngapulu-ma nganta tartartartkarra kuya nganta-wuliny karrap nyantu. Yani nganta-wula-rla. And that marluka bin come up too nganta dat lamparra na nyanuny. "Jayingka-ngantipa na ngapuku-ma, you can have 'em ngayiny daughter kujarra," kuya.

Binij. Imin warnparlk langa im na. Timpatimpak na ngawa-ma waninya. Jurlurl na waninya ngawa-ma. Pinkapinka-ma najing. Kajijirri-ma rarrarraj karu-ma nyampa-ma rarrarraj tarukap, kukijkarra. Taang mani properly way nguyina, yalungku-ma karu-ngku-ma. Marntaj.

The two of them had breasts and pubic coverings. That's how women got about in the old days. They used to wear necklaces made of seed around their necks. They used to tie them around their necks with hair string. And a bit of cloth covered their private parts.

"You two go to him. He might let the water out." He saw the two young women. The two of them went up to him. And his father-in-law came up to him too. "Give us some water and you can have my two daughters," he said.

The boy knocked the side off the tree. The water gushed out everywhere! The water spilled out all over the place. Little creeks sprang up. All of the women, children and everyone else ran and bathed and drank. That boy had deprived them of water so they were desperate. That's how the story ends!

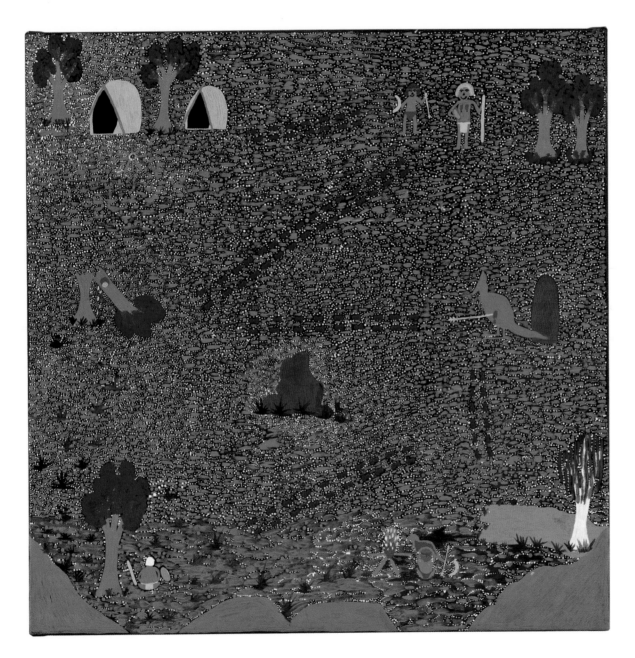

Jajurlang — The Grandmother and her Grandson
(Painting: Serena Donald, 2017)

Jajurlang — The grandmother and her grandson
told by Violet Wadrill Nanaku to Marie Japan Nangari

Yani nguwula, jajurlang nguwula yani, kajirri, karu nyanuny kaminyjarr lurta-ngarna. Jangkarni jangkarni-piya nyila-ma karu-ma. Kangani ngu nyampayirla kurlarta, an kurrupartu-kujarra karu-ngku-ma yalungku-ma. Yanani nguwula jajurlang. Kaja-ngka nguwula yanani.

Nyanuny-ju-ma jaju-ngku-ma ngawa-ma kangani pungkulung-kula, julujuluj. Murlangka ngarlaka-la kangani ngu mayingany nyanpulanguny. Yangunungku nyampa wayit, ngarlaka-la-ma kangani. Julujuluj, nyawa-ngka julujuluj kangani ngawa. Murlangka kangani kankula, pungkulung-kula jangkarni-la. Nyila-ma nyanpulany. Nyampayirla olabat wayita nyampa, mayingany nyampayirla-nguny wayita yangunungku nyampa. Ngulu kangani kuya na, kaja-ngka-ma kajijirri-lu-ma.

Yani nganta-wula well tujurt na nguwula pani makiliwarn-ma. Tujurt nguwula pani. "Warta ngarningulu jaju-ngku karlayarra murlangka-ju. Warta ngarningulu jaja-ngku. Pungka-ngali ngartin pungka-ngali! Ngarli kamparnangku kurnkurn. Pungka-ngali jaja," kuya.

Kayikayi nganta yalungku karu-ngku-ma mirlarrang-kulu jarrwaj, kurlarta-lu-kari. Yalanginyi kurrupartu-kari-lu. Yalanginyi kurrupartu-kari-lu, najing. Kalulu pungkurnangku ngarla jaja-wu ngapa-wu. Nyanuny-ma jaju-ma nganta kanya julujuluj wijkupari na.

A grandmother and grandchild were walking along — an old woman and her grandchild who was nearly ready for initiation. He was nearly an adult. That boy was carrying a shovel nose spear and a boomerang. The grandmother and grandson went along together out bush.

The grandmother was carrying water on her hip in a deep coolamon and she was carrying food on her head for the two of them. She had bush potatoes, yams and the usual things on her head, and she was carrying water on her hip in a deep coolamon. That was supposed to be for the two of them. Bush yams, potatoes … Women in the old days used to carry things like that.

Anyway, they were walking along when they startled a wallaby. The grandmother told him to hurry up and spear it. "Quick grandson! Spear some meat for us. We'll cook it with hot rocks. Kill one for us grandson," she said.

The boy chased after it and threw a shovel nose spear at it. Then another spear. And after that another spear, but he didn't hit it! Then he waited for his grandmother to give him a drink. His grandmother brought the water up close.

"Minyan jaja kula-rna pinya," kuya. "Yungka-yi ngapa jaja ngayi pungkan marta." That's Jaru, Nyininy. Im from that side na karlayarra-said that karu an kajirri nguwula.

"Ngayi marta pungan jaja ngapa yungka-yi. Kalulu kalulu jaja ngarnangku kunyjarra kunyjarra malykmalyk malykmalyk."

Nganta manani kuyangku nyangka ngawa-ma Nangari. Kuya kunyjarnani kunyjarnani kunyjarnani malykmalyk kunyjarnani. "Kalulu kalulu jaja nyangka-ngali pungku jaja kuyu. Ngarnangku yungku ngapa." Tapu manani nganta ngalyangalyakkarra nganta-nyunu kula ngarnani an water 'em manani kuya na malykmalyk malykmalyk.

Yanani nganta. Mirlarrang manani warrkuj nyila. Kurrupartu-kujarra manani warrkuj. Yanani nganta. Yanani ngu tujurt panani ngu. Tujurt ngu panani nyila-ma nyampayirla-ma wirnangpurru-ma makiliwarn-ma. Kayikayi na. Nganta palapala manani yalungku-ma karu-ngku-ma palapala palapala. Kurlarta-lu nganta pungani. Kurrupartu-kari-lu kurrupartu-kari-lu, najing. Lawara.

"Ngarna-rla kuny pungku jaja-wu ngapa-wu. Ngayu marta pungkan." Nganta liwart langa im, jaju-ma nyanuny-ma nganta imin come up ngapuku-yawung-ma julujuluj. "Jaja ngapa yungka-yi ngayi pungan. Ngarnangali ngapa-nginyi-lu-ma pungku nyila-ma, ngarin-ma," kuya.

"Sorry, granny I didn't hit it," he said in Jaru. "But give me some water, granny. I'm really thirsty." That's how Jaru and Nyininy people speak. The boy and the old woman were from the west.

"My throat is really burning, granny, give me some water. I'm waiting for you granny, sprinkle me with water."

She got the water like this, Marie. She sprinkled the water on him like this. "Wait, wait grandson, you look, shoot some meat for us! I'll give you water then," she said. She was refusing to give him any. He was trying to swallow some, but he couldn't have any because she kept just sprinkling it on him.

So he set off again. He picked up his spears and he collected his two boomerangs. And off he went. He kept going and disturbed something. He startled the same wallaby. So he took chase. The kid chased after it, chasing, chasing. He shot at it with his shovel nose spear. And with a boomerang and another. But to no avail.

"I'll wait for my grandmother to have some water. My throat's burning with thirst." He waited for her and his grandmother came up carrying the water on her hip. "Granny, give me some water, I'm thirsty! I'll try to kill a kangaroo after I've had some water," he said.

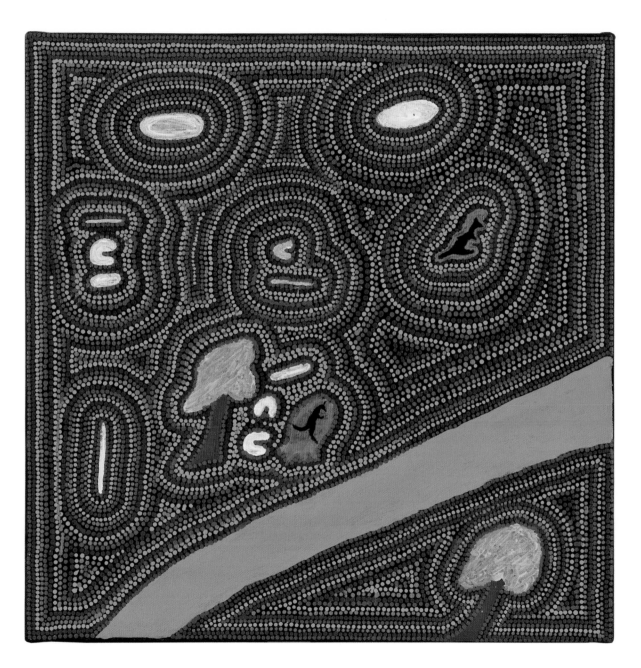

Jajurlang — The Grandmother and her Grandson
(Painting: Violet Wadrill, 2017)

"Wakurra ngarnangku kunyjarra kunyjarra." Kunyjarnani malykmalyk. Tapu ngu manani. "Malykmalyk ngurnangku kunyjarru, malykmalyk. Yangkan-ngali pungku jaja, ngarin, ngartin. Ngarnangku yungku ngapa." Marnani ngurla nyila-ma kajirri-ma jaju-ma.

Last one now. Dat karu bin kayikayi. Pinka-ma kuya na karrinya. Last one im kayikayi-ma nganta nyila-ma wirnangpurru-ma. Mirlarrang-kulu ngurla punya jarrwaj. Kurrupartu-kari-lu binij jirrpu waninya ngawa-ngka-rni dat wirnangpurru. Dat karu bin taruk langa im yirr mani outside-jirri. Kangani outside-jirri na. Pakara-yirri na kangani nyila-ma wirnangpurru-ma. Taj pani majul watjawatja ngurla pinyinyip mani warlu jiyarnani ngurla. Kamparri yanani.

Warlu-ma-rla jiyarnani. Mani kurlarr mani ngurla wirnangpurru majul-ma binij outside-ta yuwani kuya jalyi-ngka. Kuyany na kurrwararn ngurla yapakayi yuwani. Kurrwararn kuyany kurrwararn yapakayi.

Wararr ngurla-nyanta roll 'em up yuwani an karrinyani na ngurla liwart yaluwu na kajirri-wu. Ngani ngurla jaja ngu. "Jaja ngungali pinya kuyu ngari pinya. Wali punyu kula kuyarri." Ngani ngurla jaja ngu. "Ngayu kuyu punya. Wunawuna yanta-rla jaja ngan kuwarra. Kuwarra ngan nyawa. Jira ngan kuwarra jaja wuna yanta-rla."

"No I'll just sprinkle water on you," she said. She sprinkled him with water, but refused to give him any to drink. "I'm going to sprinkle you with water. You go and shoot a beast for us grandson. I'll give you some water then." That's what the old lady, his grandmother, said to him.

Finally, the boy chased after something again. This was by a river. He chased a kangaroo for the last time. He threw a spear at it and another boomerang. Suddenly the kangaroo dived into the water. The boy swam out to him and pulled it out. He took the kangaroo out of the water. He gutted it quickly, rubbed sticks together until a fire was burning. He was ahead (of the old woman who was coming up from behind).

The fire blazed. He gutted the kangaroo, putting its innards on some leaves. Then he put some small hot rocks inside its belly. The kind of small stones used for cooking.

He rolled up some fat around a rock for her and waited for the old lady. She approached him. "Granny, I've been waiting for you. I speared us some meat." The old woman went to him eagerly. "I speared the meat for us granny. Come quickly granny and swallow some. You swallow this piece. Swallow a nice fatty piece granny, come on hurry up now."

Kajirri-ma-rla rarraj yani, ngawa-ma jurlurl jurlurl jurlurl nya. "Nyawa ngan ngalu ngapa wakuwakurru na ngalu." "Ngarna ngani marntaj ngapa-ma. Binij nyawa na."

Wararr-ma yalangka-ma imin put 'em la im wumara na. Kuyangku yuwani. Karnti karnti-kujarra mani ngu kuya. Binij walyak-ma nganta mawuj-ja-ma walyak yuwanani. Kankarra ngurla-nyanta jimak punya kuyangku karnti-ku na. Binij jiyarni tampang nyila-ma kajirri-ma!

"Kuyarla karriya jaja. Ngayin taang manani ngapa-wu. Kuyala karla," kuya na. "Yu jidan jaja marntaj. Ngayin taang manani ngapa-wu. Kuya na karriya!"

Nyila-ma nganta karu-ngku-ma yalungku-ma pirtak luwani. Chuck 'em nganta kiyarni anywhere. Binij wanyjarni warrij. Wirnangpurru lajap mani yani na 'nother place-jirri na jarrwa-ngkurra na nyila-ma karu-ma. Kuya.

The old woman ran up to him spilling the water as she ran. "Drink some water now, hurry up," she said. "I've drunk enough water now," he said. "That's enough of that."

He wrapped another rock with some fat. Then he got two sticks and put the rocks on the ends and popped them in her mouth. He stuck the rocks right down her throat with the sticks. That's it — the old lady choked to death!

"You're dead now granny," he said. "That's what you get for depriving me of water. You're dead now," he said. "That's it for you now granny. You deprived me of water and now you're dead!"

Then the boy disposed of his grandmother and upped and left. He slung the kangaroo over his shoulder then went to another place where there were lots of people. That's how it was.

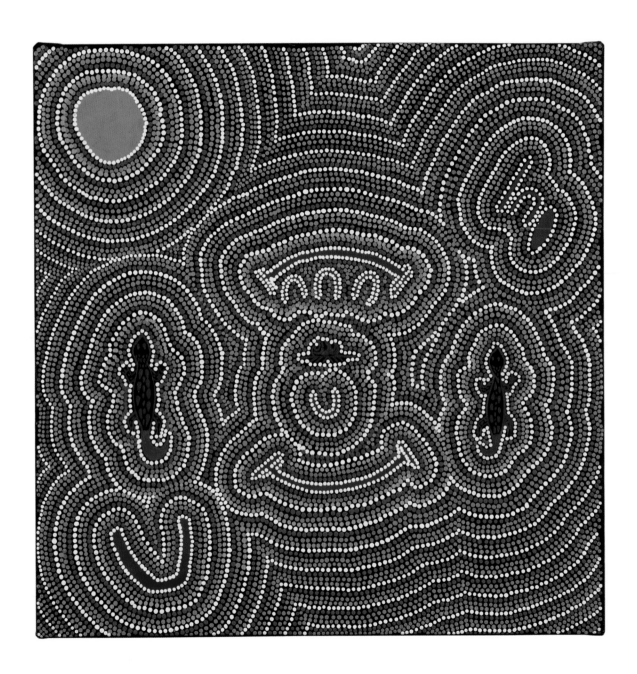

Jampurra — The Cry Baby
(Painting: Violet Wadrill, 2017)

Jampurra — The cry baby

told by Violet Wadrill Nanaku

Nyawa-ma-rnangku-rla malu yurrk yaluwu na karu-wu. Karu-ma nyila-ma Jampurra. Jampurra-la-ngarna im ngamayi-wu ngayiny-ku Dreamtime story Jampurra-ma. Nyila-ma karu-ma ngulu yingkij manani kuyangku-ma. Kula-lu panani ngulu yingkij panani kuyangku. Nurrk ngulu jayingani. Nyantu-ma lungkarra lungani ngu.

"Warta nyawa-kata nyalu parra ngama walu jijal-jawung jijal-jawung-ma tal parra!" marnani nyila-ma karu-ma, Jampurra-ma, Jampurra-ngarna yini. "Nyawa-kata nyalu ngama walu kuwaru-ma tal parra!"

"Warta karrarra karrarra karrarra! Nyampa-wu-ja-nta panana? Nyila-ma karrarra, lungkarrapkaji ngu, wanyjarra-lu, lungkarrap-kaji!"

Yalanginyi-ma-rla nganta wajawajarra ngulu karrinyani. Kurlpakurlpap-ma wumara jiwajiwarrp na ngulu yanani karrinyani ngulu kurlpakurlpap. Nyila ngu karu ngu nganta jintapa-kari-lu-ma yingyingarn jiyarnani kuyangku-ma. "Warta nyawa-kata nyalu walu jijal-jawung jijal-jawung-ma tal parra ngama. Walu kunangkuta kunangkuta-ma tal parra."

I'm going to tell you a story about a child. The child was called Jampurra. This story is from my mother's country. It is Tommy Dodd (Topsy Dodd Ngarnjal's first husband), Ida Malyik and Daisy Jalpngarri's country. They teased that kid mercilessly. They weren't hitting him hard, just jabbing him. They were just prodding him. But it made him cry.

"Hey Mummy — they're calling me 'grassy head'!" This is what the kid Jampurra said. Jampurra was his name. "Hey Mummy — they're calling me 'pointy head'!".

"Hey stop it you mob, leave him be! Why do you mob insist on punching him? Stop it, he's a cry baby, leave him alone — he's a sook!" said his mother.

After that, they played nicely together for a bit. They came together in a group, heaping up stones. But another kid started pushing and shoving him. "Hey mummy this one's calling me 'grassy head'! Hey mum he's calling me 'scabby head'!" he said.

"Karrarra karrarra nyila-ma karu-ma nomo parra-lu kuyarra. Wanyjarra-lu lungkarrap-kaji ngu ngalyapa nyila-ma wanyjarra-lu. Karrinyani ngulu yalanginyi-ma pirrkappirrkapkarra nyampa-kayirnikayirni nganta-lu manani wumara nyampa kurlpapkurlpap yuwanani yalanginyi-ma. "Warta nyawa-kata nyalu ngama walu jijal-jawung jijal-jawung-ma tal parra, nyila na karu jijal-jawung. Marntaj purrp that much na.

Ngurra Jijaljawung-ngarna ngamayi-wu ngayiny-ku nguyina Dreamtime stori nyawa-ma jarrakap nyarrulunguny. Karlangkarla murlanginyi karlarnimpa kankula. Putjuwarriny, marntaj.

"Hey stop it, don't hit that kid!" she said, "Just leave him alone — he's a sook who won't stop crying — leave him be." After that they were sitting around building something or other by heaping up stones. "Hey mummy they're calling me 'grassy head'!" And so it went on!

This is a Dreamtime story about my mother's country from Nawurla country which they told me. It's west of Kalkaringi in the eastern part of Limbunya Station around Putjuwarriny and Turtungkayak (Number 18 Bore).

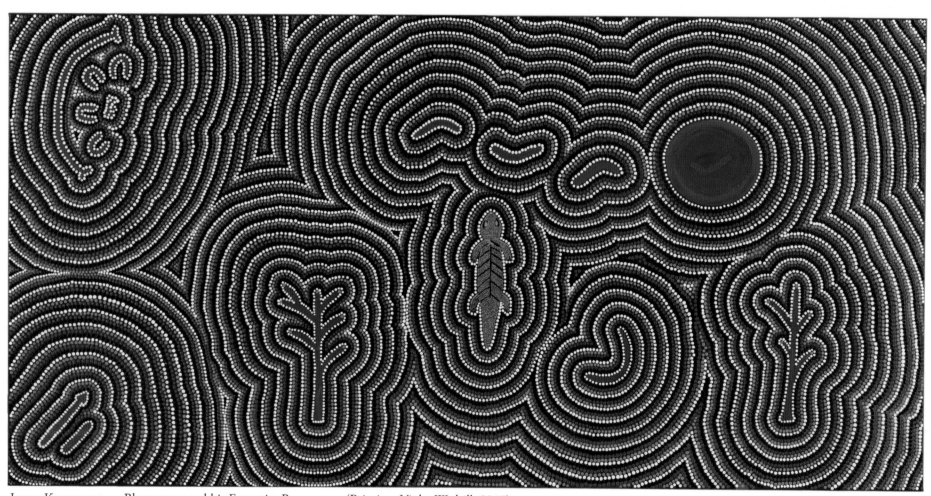

Luma Kurrupartu — Bluetongue and his Favourite Boomerang (Painting: Violet Wadrill, 2017)

Luma kurrupartu — The bluetongue and his favourite boomerang

told by Violet Wadrill Nanaku

Bluetongue-ma nyila-ma nganayirla-ma. Yuwani ngu warntarrija kurrupartu-ma, nyampayirla-lu-ma luma-ngku-ma. Yikili-ngurlu yuwani. Yuwani ngu ngawa-ngka kanyjurra Lutu-ngka. Jirrpu waninya. Ngawa-ngka japurr, jirrpu ngu yuwani ngawa-ngka. Nyangani ngurla warlakap. Warlakap ngurla nyangani wanyjingurlu yanani yanani ngu. Kurlarra yanani ngu. Palangari-yirri yalangkurra. Karrap ngurla nyangani. "Murlangurlu murlangurlu na ngurna yuwani-ma." "Wanyjika-rna yuwani?" Ngurla nyangani kuyangku-ma, "Wanyjirniny-pa-rna yuwani wanyjirniny-pa-rna-rla tarrjal mani, nyamu-rna warntarrija yuwani?"

This is a story about Bluetongue. Bluetongue threw a boomerang a long way (across a plain). He threw it into a waterhole called Lutu and it sank down. It went into the water when he threw it in. He searched for it everywhere. He kept searching for it going from this place to that place. He went south to the black soil plain. He was looking around for it there. "It was from here that I threw it," he thought. "So where did it end up?" He wanted to go back to the same place where he threw it from. He kept searching for it muttering, "Which way did I throw it? Where's the mark it would have made upon landing?"

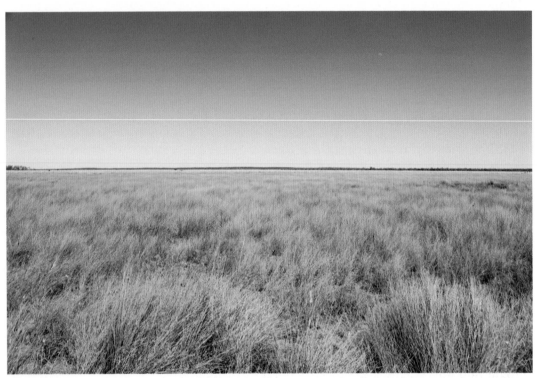

Blacksoil plain near Lutu on Limbunya Station (Photo: Penny Smith, 2015)

Yanani ngu yalangkurra. Nyangani ngurla kuyangku-ma murlangurlu na, "Nyawa na nyawarniny nyawa ngurna yuwani-ma." "Kula-rna paraj pungana. Wanyjika wayi-rna yuwani yikili?" "Ngurna waninya nyawa wanyjika waku maitbi kayirrak. Yuwani ngurna ngapuku-la maitbi, kanyjurra murlangka." Lutu nyila-ma ngawa-ma kanyjurra-ma. Ngurla nyangani kuyangku-ma, lawara lungkarrap na ngurla karrinyani.

Yalanginyi-ma yanani ngu pina-ngkurra-rni karrap ngurla nyangani. Pina-ngurlu-rni, yanani ngu kuya kalurirrp, kaarnimpal-said. Kalurirrip yanani ngu. Nyangani ngurla lawara. Kula paraj pungani. Karlayarra-said kurlarrak yanani ngu. Nyangani ngurla lawara. "Kula-rna paraj pungku. Ngajik ngurna yanani wanyjika-rna yuwani?"

Nyangani ngu-rla majul-lu-ma patawarn-tu patawarn-tu patawarn-tu najing yalanginyi-ma lawara. Lungkarra na ngurla lungani. Miyikarra manani ngunyunu, kuyany-ma ngapanyji-ma. Nyamu-rla lungkarrap-ma karrinyani.

Yanani ngu pina-ngkurra-rni karrap ngurla nyangani. "Wanyjirniny-pa-rna yuwani?" Mirriwantuk-kulu karrap. "Wanyjika-rna yuwani? Marulu ngurna nyila-ma kurrupartu-ma. Kamparrajang." Nyawarra dijan nyampayirla yijarni nyawa. Marulu-wu-ma yaluwu-ma. Lungkarrap ngurla lungani. Lungkarrap-ma-rla karrinyani kuya.

He went to another place. He kept looking around, then he exclaimed, "That's it, I threw it this way. But I can't find it. Oh why did I throw it such a long way away? Well maybe it is north of here," he said. "Maybe I threw it in the water, right down here." Lutu is a deep waterhole. He looked everywhere for it there, but to no avail and so he sat there crying about it.

Then Bluetongue went to the same place where he threw the boomerang and looked there. And from the same place, he walked about on the east side of the plain. He walked about there and looked for it everywhere, but no luck. He couldn't find it. From the west side of the plain, he went south. He looked everywhere for it. "I won't be able to find it," he said. "I've been going about for ages, oh where did I throw it?"

Bluetongue kept looking around bravely without crying, but then it was all too much. He burst into tears over his boomerang. He wiped away his tears from his eyes. He made black stripes under his eyes when he was crying about it.

Bluetongue went back to the same place and looked for it there. "Which way did I throw it?" he asked himself. He looked into the distance with his hand on his brow. "Oh where did I throw it?" he thought. "That's my favourite boomerang. I had it for such a long time." This is true! That was his favourite boomerang. He sat there crying over it.

Kayiliyin-jirri yanani ngu kayirrak. Nyangku-nta-nga nyila-ma palangari-ma. Kula yapawurru. Nyamu-rla nyangani-ma. Kaarnimpal-la-said ngurla nyangani. Yalanginyi-ma yanani wart kurlarra-nganang. Nyamu-nga yuwani kurlayirra-tu wantarrija kayirranganang. Yalanginyi-ma karlayarra-said yanani ngu kurlarrak nyangani ngurla karrap kurlaniyin-tu. "Lawara wanyjika wayi-rna yuwani? Wayi-rna yuwani ngawa-ngka kanyjurra japurr?"

Nyangani ngurla karrinya na. Yani, kurlartarti-ngkurra yalangkurra. Kutij karrinya, yalangka-ma kurlartarti-la-ma. Wanyjarni ngu dat kurlartarti kutij. Nyantu na nyamu-ma karrinya puwarraja kutij. Yani ngu, yalangkurra ngawa-ngkurra-ma kanyjurra Lutu-ngkurra-ma. Kuya na karlarrak karrinya. Karrakarrapkarra ngurla nyangani lawara. Yani nyila na, kurlartarti jeya na ngawa-ngka kutij. Nyila-ma nyantu na. Puwarraj puwarraja. Nyila-ma kurlartarti-ma nyantu.

Bluetongue looked for it at Lutu and there he stayed. (He was tired but realised he had thrown into the water). He went to a bush orange tree. He stood by the tree. Then the tree disappeared and he became the tree. That's him now — Bluetongue had become a Dreaming tree. Bluetongue had gone down to the water's edge at Lutu. To the place on the west side. He had kept looking there, but it was all in vain. He had gone there and now there is a bush orange standing by the water's edge. That's Bluetongue there. He's now a Dreaming tree. He had transformed into the bush orange tree.

Marntaj. Yeah ngayiny-ku ngamayi-wu, ngayiny-ku jawiji-wu, nyila-ma nguyina, nyampayirla-ma puwarraj-ma nyila-ma.

Bluetongue went from the north and back north again. You should see the black soil plain! It's not small! He was looking around for it this way and that. He looked for it on the east side. Then Bluetongue went south, facing east to west, because he threw the boomerang from the south. Then from the west side, he went south looking for it. "I can't find it — oh where did I throw it?" he cried. "Oh did I throw it into Lutu?"

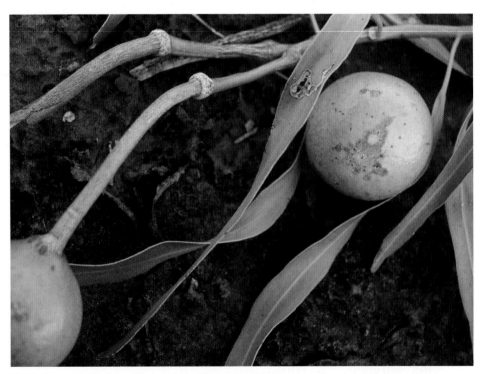

Fruit from a *kurlartarti* (Capparis umbonata)

That's the end of the story. That Dreaming is my mother's and mother's father's.

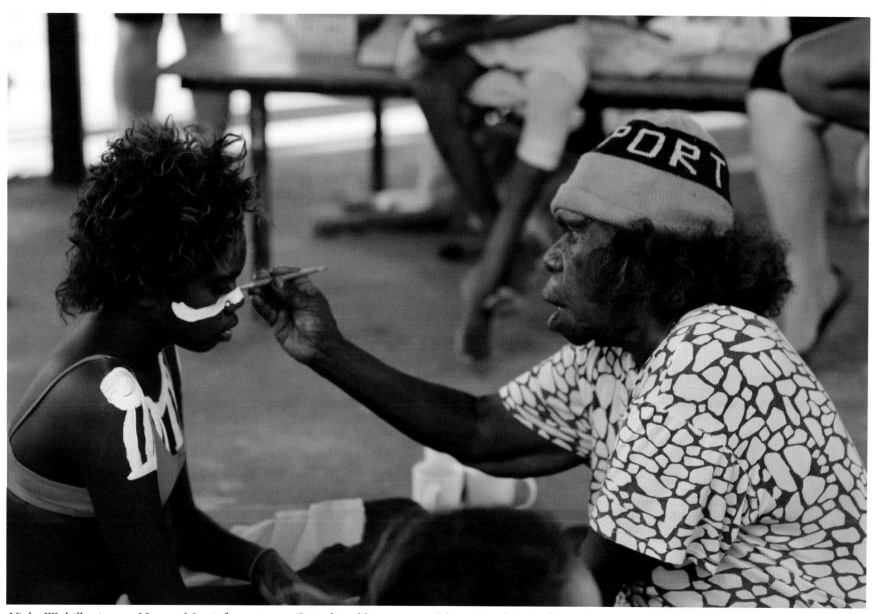

Violet Wadrill paints up Nazeera Morris for wajarra, a Gurindji public ceremony (Photo: Brenda L Croft, 2015)

Story sources

Title	Author	Year	Recording, Transcription and Translation	Recording Number
Introduction statement	Violet Wadrill	2007	Felicity Meakins	FM07_a01_1b
Karungkarni — The place of the children	Violet Wadrill	2010	Felicity Meakins	FM10_30_1a
Yimaruk — Animal spirits	Biddy Wavehill	2009	Felicity Meakins	FM09_a122
Wartiwarti karu — Born left-handed	Violet Wadrill	2010	Felicity Meakins	FM10_a143
Punyu mangarri ngarturr-ku — Good foods for pregnant women	Biddy Wavehill	2009	Felicity Meakins	FM09_a122
Kiliny — Goanna with eggs	Violet Wadrill	2009	Felicity Meakins	FM09_a123
Jamut — Bush turkey	Violet Wadrill	2009	Felicity Meakins	FM09_a123
Yiparrartu — Emu	Violet Wadrill	2009	Felicity Meakins	FM09_a123
Narrinyjila — Turtle	Violet Wadrill	2009	Felicity Meakins	FM09_a123
Wintuk — Bush stone-curlew	Violet Wadrill	2009	Felicity Meakins	FM11_a167
Jungkuwurru — Echidna	Violet Wadrill	2009	Felicity Meakins	FM09_a123
Ngapuk ngarin — Smelling cooking meat	Violet Wadrill	2009	Felicity Meakins	FM09_a123
Ngamayi kamparnup — Treating mothers after birth	Violet Wadrill	2010	Felicity Meakins	FM10_a149
Ngapulu kamparnup — Promoting milk	Violet Wadrill	2012	Felicity Meakins	FM12_33_1
Karu kamparnup –Treatments using termite mound	Violet Wadrill	2008	Felicity Meakins	FM08_a085
Karu kamparnup –Treatments using termite mound	Biddy Wavehill	2009	Felicity Meakins	FM09_a143

Title	Author	Year	Recording, Transcription and Translation	Recording Number
Warra karu parntawurru — Looking after babies' backs	Violet Wadrill	2008	Felicity Meakins	FM07_a050
Purntunarri kamparnup — Treating older babies	Connie Ngarmeiya	2010	Felicity Meakins	FM11_31_3a
Yarnanti rarraj-ku — A charm for running	Dandy Danbayarri	2007	Lauren Campbell	R00891_05
Ngarrka karu-walija — Introducing children to country and ancestors	Violet Wadrill	2018	Felicity Meakins	FM18_a511
Manyanyi and marlarn — Bush vicks and red river gum	Biddy Wavehill	2010	Felicity Meakins	FM10_a143
Yarnanti kulykulyu-wu — A charm for colds	Dandy Danbayarri	2007	Lauren Campbell	R00891_03
Punyukkaji kulykulyu-wu — Cures for colds	Kitty Mintawurr, Biddy Wavehill	2009	Felicity Meakins	FM09_14_3
Yirrijkaji, wariyili and partiki	Violet Wadrill, Biddy Wavehill	1998	Erika Charola	Video
Jikirrij — Willie-wagtail	Violet Wadrill	2014	Felicity Meakins	FM14_a226
Wirnangpurru — Kangaroo	Violet Wadrill	2009	Felicity Meakins	FM09_a123
Warrija kirrawa — The crocodile and goanna	Violet Wadrill	2010	Felicity Meakins	FM10_23_2a
Ngarlking karu — The greedy child	Violet Wadrill	2010	Felicity Meakins	FM10_a155
Jajurlang — The grandmother and her grandson	Violet Wadrill	2010	Felicity Meakins	FM10_30_2a
Jampurra — The Cry Baby	Violet Wadrill	2012	Felicity Meakins	FM12_34_1a
Luma kurrupartu — The bluetongue and his favourite boomerang	Violet Wadrill	2009	Felicity Meakins	FM10_23_1a

If you would like to know more about
Spinifex Press, write to us for a free catalogue,
visit our website and social media pages or email us
for further information on how to subscribe
to our monthly newsletter.

Spinifex Press
PO Box 105
Mission Beach QLD 4852
Australia

Orders:
PO Box 5270
North Geelong Vic 3215
Australia

www.spinifexpress.com.au
women@spinifexpress.com.au